ABC OF
LEARNING AND TEACHING IN MEDICINE

Edited by

PETER CANTILLON
Senior lecturer in medical informatics and medical education,
National University of Ireland, Galway, Republic of Ireland

LINDA HUTCHINSON
Director of education and workforce development and consultant paediatrician,
University Hospital Lewisham

and

DIANA WOOD
Director of medical education, University of Cambridge School of Clinical Medicine,
Addenbrookes Hospital, Cambridge

BMJ
Books

A 031933

W18

First published in 2003
Second impression 2003
Third impression 2004
by BMJ Publishing Group Ltd, BMA House, Tavistock Square,
London WC1H 9JR

www.bmjbooks.com

British Library Cataloguing in Publication Data
A catalogue record for this book is available from the British Library

ISBN 07279 16785

Typeset by BMJ Electronic Production
Printed and bound in Spain by GraphyCems, Navarra   .
Cover Image shows a stethoscope for listening to sounds within the body
With permission from Colin Cuthbert/Science Photo Library

A 031933

ABC OF
LEARNING AND TEACHING IN MEDICINE

£17.28

Contents

Contributors

Peter Cantillon
Senior lecturer in medical informatics and medical education, National University of Ireland, Galway, Republic of Ireland

Richard Farrow
Director of problem based learning at the Peninsula Medical School at the Universities of Exeter and Plymouth

Jill Gordon
Associate professor in the department of medical education at the University of Sydney, Australia

Linda Hutchinson
Director of education and workforce development and consultant paediatrician, University Hospital Lewisham, London

David Jaques
Independent consultant in learning and teaching in higher education

Carol Jollie
Project officer in the skills enhancement project for the Camden Primary Care Trust at St Pancras Hospital, London

David M Kaufman
Director of the Learning and Instructional Development Centre at Simon Fraser University, Burnaby, British Columbia, Canada

Judy McKimm
Head of curriculum development at Imperial College School of Medicine, London and an educational consultant

Jill Morrison
Professor of general practice and deputy associate dean for education at Glasgow University

John J Norcini
President and chief executive officer of the Foundation for Advancement of International Medical Education and Research, Philadelphia, Pennsylvania

David Prideaux
Professor and head of the Office of Medical Education in the School of Medicine at Flinders University, Adelaide, Australia

Lambert W T Schuwirth
Assistant professor in the department of educational development and research at the University of Maastricht in the Netherlands

Sydney Smee
Manager of the Medical Council of Canada's qualifying examination part II, in Ottawa, Canada

John Spencer
General practitioner and professor of medical education in primary health care at the University of Newcastle upon Tyne

Cees P M van der Vleuten
Professor and chair in the department of educational development and research at the University of Maastricht in the Netherlands

Diana Wood
Director of medical education, University of Cambridge School of Clinical Medicine, Addenbrookes Hospital, Cambridge

Preface

Although we would never allow a patient to be treated by an untrained doctor or nurse, we often tolerate professional training being delivered by untrained teachers. Traditionally students were expected to absorb most of their medical education by attending timetabled lectures and ward-rounds, moving rapidly from one subject to the next in a crowded curriculum. Our junior doctors learnt by watching their seniors in between endless menial tasks. In recent years the importance of active, self directed learning in higher education has been recognised. Outcome led structured programmes for trainees are being developed in the face of reduced working hours for both the learners and teachers. These all present new challenges for teachers in medicine of all levels of seniority.

Throughout the world there is great interest in developing a set of qualifications for medical teachers, both at the elementary "teaching the teacher" level and as part of progressive modular programmes leading to formal certification. In addition to acquiring new qualifications and standards, teachers also need access to literature resources that describe essential components in medical education and supply tips and ideas for teaching.

This ABC began as an expressed wish of the BMJ to publish an introductory and accessible text on medical education. It grew into a book covering the more generic topics of learning and teaching in medicine with the aim of illustrating how educational theory and research underpins the practicalities of teaching and learning. The editors invited an international group of authors on the basis of their acknowledged expertise in the particular topics assigned to them. Each chapter was edited and illustrated to ensure maximum accessibility for readers and subsequently peer reviewed by two educational experts. Their suggestions have been incorporated into the finished book.

The *ABC of Learning and Teaching in Medicine* would not have been possible without the tireless support of BMJ editorial staff, Julia Thompson, Eleanor Lines, Sally Carter, and Naomi Wilkinson. We would also like to thank Professor Paul O' Neill and Dr Ed Peile for their excellent and timely peer reviews for each of the chapters. Finally we would very much welcome comments and suggestions about this ABC from its most important reviewers, you the readers.

PC, DW, LH

1 Applying educational theory in practice

David M Kaufman

How many times have we as teachers been confronted with situations in which we really were not sure what to do? We "flew by the seat of our pants," usually doing with our learners what had been done with us. It would be useful to be able to turn to a set of guiding principles based on evidence, or at least on long term successful experience.

Fortunately, a body of theory exists that can inform practice. An unfortunate gap between academics and practitioners, however, has led to a perception of theory as belonging to an "ivory tower" and not relevant to practice. Yet the old adage that "there is nothing more practical than a good theory" still rings true today. This chapter describes several educational theories and guiding principles and then shows how these could be applied to three case studies relating to the "real world."

Adult learning theory

Malcolm Knowles introduced the term "andragogy" to North America, defining it as "the art and science of helping adults learn." Andragogy is based on five assumptions—about how adults learn and their attitude towards and motivation for learning.

Knowles later derived seven principles of andragogy. Most theorists agree that andragogy is not really a theory of adult learning, but they regard Knowles' principles as guidelines on how to teach learners who tend to be at least somewhat independent and self directed. His principles can be summarised as follows:
- Establish an effective learning climate, where learners feel safe and comfortable expressing themselves
- Involve learners in mutual planning of relevant methods and curricular content
- Involve learners in diagnosing their own needs—this will help to trigger internal motivation
- Encourage learners to formulate their own learning objectives—this gives them more control of their learning
- Encourage learners to identify resources and devise strategies for using the resources to achieve their objectives
- Support learners in carrying out their learning plans
- Involve learners in evaluating their own learning—this can develop their skills of critical reflection.

Self directed learning

Self directed learning can be viewed as a method of organising teaching and learning in which the learning tasks are largely within the learners' control (as with the adult learning principles described above).

It can also be viewed as a goal towards which learners strive so that they become empowered to accept personal responsibility for their own learning, personal autonomy, and individual choice. Success in the first view would lead to attaining the second.

Philip Candy identified in the literature about 100 traits associated with self direction, which he synthesised as the ability to be methodical and disciplined; logical and analytical; collaborative and interdependent; curious, open, creative, and motivated; persistent and responsible; confident and competent at learning; and reflective and self aware.

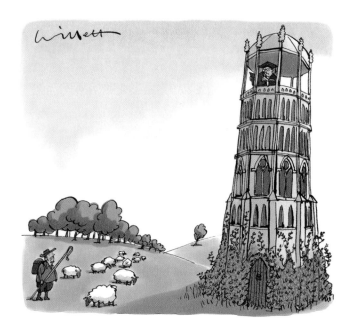

Andragogy—five assumptions about adult learning
- Adults are independent and self directing
- They have accumulated a great deal of experience, which is a rich resource for learning
- They value learning that integrates with the demands of their everyday life
- They are more interested in immediate, problem centred approaches than in subject centred ones
- They are more motivated to learn by internal drives than by external ones

---

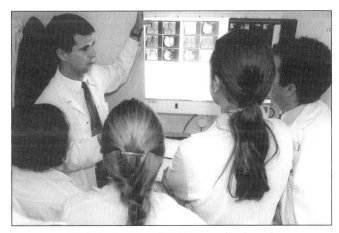

Learners need to feel safe and comfortable expressing themselves

---

Self directed learning
- Organising teaching and learning so that learning is within the learners' control
- A goal towards which learners strive so that they become able to accept responsibility for their own learning

How do we develop these traits in our learners? Most importantly, learners must have the opportunity to develop and practise skills that directly improve self directed learning. These skills include asking questions, critically appraising new information, identifying their own knowledge and skill gaps, and reflecting critically on their learning process and outcomes.

Self efficacy

According to Albert Bandura, people's judgments of their own ability to deal with different situations is central to their actions. These actions include what they choose to do, how much effort they invest in activities, how long they persist in the face of adversity, and whether they approach the tasks anxiously or assuredly.

These judgments, called "self efficacy," may or may not be accurate, but they arise from four main information sources. In decreasing order of their strength, these sources are: performance attainments, observations of other people, verbal persuasion, and physiological state. Successes raise our self efficacy, while failures lower it. Failures are particularly likely to lower our self efficacy if they occur early in the learning process and are not due to lack of effort or difficult situations.

Observing other people similar to us performing successfully can strengthen our beliefs that we can perform similar tasks, especially when the tasks are unfamiliar. Verbal persuasion from a credible source also can help.

Finally, we (both teachers and learners) need to re-interpret our anxiety or nervousness in difficult situations as excitement or anticipation, rather than as an ominous sign of vulnerability.

Constructivism

Constructivism has important implications for teaching and learning. Firstly, the teacher is viewed not as a transmitter of knowledge but as a guide who facilitates learning. Secondly, as learning is based on prior knowledge, teachers should provide learning experiences that expose inconsistencies between students' current understandings and their new experiences. Thirdly, teachers should engage students in their learning in an active way, using relevant problems and group interaction. Fourthly, if new knowledge is to be actively acquired, sufficient time must be provided for in-depth examination of new experiences.

Reflective practice

The theory of reflective practice is attributed primarily to Donald Schön, whose work is based on the study of a range of professions. He argues that formal theory acquired through professional preparation is often not useful to the solution of the real life "messy, indeterminate" problems of practice.

Schön labels professionals' automatic ways of practising as professional "zones of mastery"—that is, areas of competence. Unexpected events or surprises trigger two kinds of reflection.

The first, "reflection in action," occurs immediately. It is the ability to learn and develop continually by creatively applying current and past experiences and reasoning to unfamiliar events while they are occurring. The second, "reflection on action," occurs later. It is a process of thinking back on what happened in a past situation, what may have contributed to the unexpected event, whether the actions taken were appropriate, and how this situation may affect future practice.

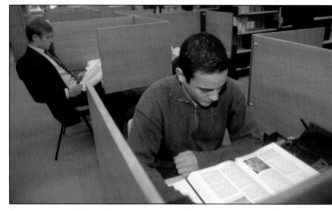

Learners should identify their own knowledge gaps and critically appraise new information

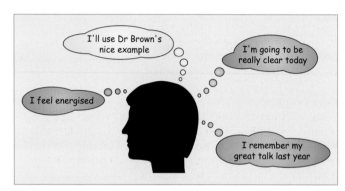

Teachers and learners need to view any anxiety or nervousness in difficult situations as excitement or anticipation

Self efficacy—roles for the teacher

- Modelling or demonstration
- Setting a clear goal or image of the desired outcome
- Providing basic knowledge and skills needed as the foundation for the task
- Providing guided practice with corrective feedback
- Giving students the opportunity to reflect on their learning

The primary idea of constructivism is that learners "construct" their own knowledge on the basis of what they already know. This theory posits that learning is active, rather than passive, with learners making judgments about when and how to modify their knowledge

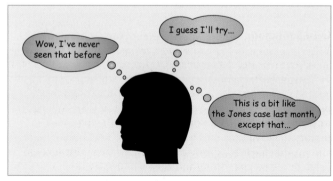

"Reflection in action"

Through the process of reflecting both "in practice" and "on practice," practitioners continually reshape their approaches and develop "wisdom" or "artistry" in their practice. Activities such as debriefing with peers or learners, seeking feedback from learners on a regular basis, and keeping a journal can provide vehicles for reflective practice.

Converting theory into practice

Each of the educational theories presented here can guide our teaching practices. Some theories will be more helpful than others in particular contexts. However, several principles also emerge from these theories, and these can provide helpful guidance for medical educators.

Three cases studies
The boxes (right) describe three "real world" case studies representing situations encountered in medical education settings. The educational theories described above, and the principles which emerge from them, can guide us in solving the problems posed in these three cases.

Case 1 solution
You could present an interactive lecture on the autonomic nervous system. You could distribute a notetaking guide. This would contain key points, space for written notes, and two key multiple choice or "short answer" questions requiring higher level thinking (principle 1, see box above). You could stop twice during the lecture and ask the students to discuss their response to each question with their neighbours (principles 1, 3, and 5). A show of hands would determine the class responses to the question (checking for understanding) and you could then give the correct answer (principle 5). Finally, you could assign a learning issue for the students to research in their own time (principle 4).

Case 2 solution
You could assign the students to small groups of four to six, and ask each group to submit two case studies describing clinical ethics issues in their local hospitals (principles 1 and 2). The ethics theory and approach needed to analyse these cases could be prepared by experts and presented on a website in advance of the sessions (principles 4, 5). The first of the six blocks of two hours could be used to discuss the material on the website and clarify any misunderstandings (principle 5). You could then show the students how to work though a case, with participation by the class (principle 7). The other five blocks could then be used for each small group to work through some of the cases prepared earlier, followed by a debriefing session with the whole class (principles 5 and 6).

Case 3 solution
You could first invite the registrar to observe you with patients, and do a quick debrief at the end of the day (principles 2, 6, and 7). With help from you, she could then develop her own learning goals, based on the certification requirements and perceived areas of weakness (principles 1, 3, and 4). These goals would provide the framework for assessing the registrar's performance with patients (principles 5, 6). You could observe and provide feedback (principle 5). Finally, the registrar could begin to see patients alone and keep a journal (written or electronic) in which she records the results of "reflection on practice" (principle 6). She could also record in her journal the personal learning issues arising from her patients, could conduct self directed learning on these, and could document

Seven principles to guide teaching practice
1 The learner should be an active contributor to the educational process
2 Learning should closely relate to understanding and solving real life problems
3 Learners' current knowledge and experience are critical in new learning situations and need to be taken into account
4 Learners should be given the opportunity and support to use self direction in their learning
5 Learners should be given opportunities and support for practice, accompanied by self assessment and constructive feedback from teachers and peers
6 Learners should be given opportunities to reflect on their practice; this involves analysing and assessing their own performance and developing new perspectives and options
7 Use of role models by medical educators has a major impact on learners. As people often teach the way they were taught, medical educators should model these educational principles with their students and junior doctors. This will help the next generation of teachers and learners to become more effective and should lead to better care for patients

Case 1: Teaching basic science
You have been asked to give a lecture on the autonomic nervous system to a first year medical class of 120 students. This has traditionally been a difficult subject for the class, particularly as it has not been explicitly covered by faculty in the problem based anatomy course. You wonder how you can make this topic understandable to the class in a 50-minute lecture.

Case 2: Ethics education
You are a member of a course committee in the department of internal medicine, which is charged with the task of integrating the topic of ethics into the third year medicine rotation. Your committee has been given six blocks of two hours over a 12 week period. You wonder how to make the material engaging, understandable, and useful to the students.

Case 3: General practice training
You are the trainer for a first year registrar in her first year of a general practice training programme. Your practice is so busy that you have very little time to spend with her. You wonder how you can contribute to providing a valuable learning experience for your trainee.

her findings in the journal (principles 1, 4, and 6). You could provide feedback on the journal (principle 5). If practical, the cohort of registrars could communicate via the internet to discuss their insights and experiences (principle 6).

Conclusions

This article has attempted to show how the gap between educational theory and practice can be bridged. By using teaching and learning methods based on educational theories and derived principles, medical educators will become more effective teachers. This will enhance the development of knowledge, skills, and positive attitudes in their learners, and improve the next generation of teachers. Ultimately, this should result in better trained doctors who provide an even higher level of patient care and improved patient outcomes.

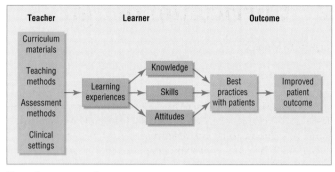

From theory to practice

Further reading

- Bandura A. *Social foundations of thought and action: a social cognitive theory.* Englewood Cliffs, NJ: Prentice-Hall, 1986.
- Candy PC. *Self-direction for lifelong learning: a comprehensive guide to theory and practice.* San Francisco: Jossey-Bass, 1991.
- Kaufman DM, Mann KV, Jennett P. *Teaching and learning in medical education: how theory can inform practice.* London: Association for the Study of Medical Education, 2000. (Monograph.)
- Knowles MS and Associates. *Andragogy in action: applying modern principles of adult learning.* San Francisco: Jossey-Bass, 1984.
- Schön DA. *Educating the reflective practitioner: toward a new design for teaching and learning in the professions.* San Francisco: Jossey-Bass, 1987.

2 Curriculum design

David Prideaux

The curriculum represents the expression of educational ideas in practice. The word curriculum has its roots in the Latin word for track or race course. From there it came to mean course of study or syllabus. Today the definition is much wider and includes all the planned learning experiences of a school or educational institution.

The curriculum must be in a form that can be communicated to those associated with the learning institution, should be open to critique, and should be able to be readily transformed into practice. The curriculum exists at three levels: what is planned for the students, what is delivered to the students, and what the students experience.

A curriculum is the result of human agency. It is underpinned by a set of values and beliefs about what students should know and how they come to know it. The curriculum of any institution is often contested and problematic. Some people may support a set of underlying values that are no longer relevant. This is the so called sabretoothed curriculum, which is based on the fable of the cave dwellers who continued to teach about hunting the sabretoothed tiger long after it became extinct. In contemporary medical education it is argued that the curriculum should achieve a "symbiosis" with the health services and communities in which the students will serve. The values that underlie the curriculum should enhance health service provision. The curriculum must be responsive to changing values and expectations in education if it is to remain useful.

Elements of a curriculum

If curriculum is defined more broadly than syllabus or course of study then it needs to contain more than mere statements of content to be studied. A curriculum has at least four important elements: content; teaching and learning strategies; assessment processes; and evaluation processes.

The process of defining and organising these elements into a logical pattern is known as curriculum design. Curriculum writers have tried to place some order or rationality on the process of designing a curriculum by advocating models.

There are two main types: prescriptive models, which indicate what curriculum designers should do; and descriptive models, which purport to describe what curriculum designers actually do. A consideration of these models assists in understanding two additional key elements in curriculum design: statements of intent and context.

Prescriptive models

Prescriptive models are concerned with the ends rather than the means of a curriculum. One of the more well known examples is the "objectives model," which arose from the initial work of Ralph Tyler in 1949. According to this model, four important questions are used in curriculum design.

The first question, about the "purposes" to be obtained, is the most important one. The statements of purpose have become known as "objectives," which should be written in terms of changed behaviour among learners that can be easily measured. This was interpreted very narrowly by some people and led to the specification of verbs that are acceptable and those that are unacceptable when writing the so called

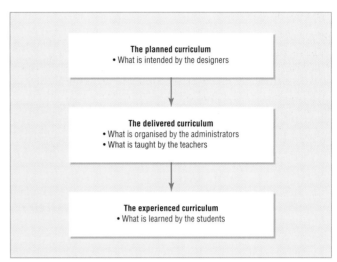

Three levels of a curriculum

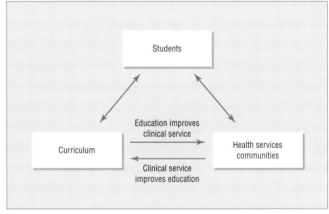

"Symbiosis" necessary for a curriculum. From Bligh J et al (see "Further reading" box)

Curriculum models

Prescriptive models
- What curriculum designers should do
- How to create a curriculum

Descriptive models
- What curriculum designers actually do
- What a curriculum covers

Objectives model—four important questions*
- What educational purposes should the institution seek to attain?
- What educational experiences are likely to attain the purposes?
- How can these educational experiences be organised effectively?
- How can we determine whether these purposes are being attained?

*Based on Tyler R. *Basic principles of curriculum and instruction.* Chicago: Chicago University Press, 1949

"behavioural objectives." Once defined, the objectives are then used to determine the other elements of the curriculum (content; teaching and learning strategies; assessment; and evaluation).

This model has attracted some criticism—for example, that it is difficult and time consuming to construct behavioural objectives. A more serious criticism is that the model restricts the curriculum to a narrow range of student skills and knowledge that can be readily expressed in behavioural terms. Higher order thinking, problem solving, and processes for acquiring values may be excluded because they cannot be simply stated in behavioural terms. As a result of such criticism the objectives model has waned in popularity. The importance of being clear about the purpose of the curriculum is well accepted.

More recently, another prescriptive model of curriculum design has emerged. "Outcomes based education" is similar in many respects to the objectives model and again starts from a simple premise—the curriculum should be defined by the outcomes to be obtained by students. Curriculum design proceeds by working "backwards" from outcomes to the other elements (content; teaching and learning experiences; assessment; and evaluation).

The use of outcomes is becoming more popular in medical education, and this has the important effect of focusing curriculum designers on what the students will do rather than what the staff do. Care should be taken, however, to focus only on "significant and enduring" outcomes. An exclusive concern with specific competencies or precisely defined knowledge and skills to be acquired may result in the exclusion of higher order content that is important in preparing medical professionals.

Although debate may continue about the precise form of these statements of intent (as they are known), they constitute an important element of curriculum design. It is now well accepted that curriculum designers will include statements of intent in the form of both broad curriculum aims and more specific objectives in their plans. Alternatively, intent may be expressed in terms of broad and specific curriculum outcomes. The essential function of these statements is to require curriculum designers to consider clearly the purposes of what they do in terms of the effects and impact on students.

Descriptive models

An enduring example of a descriptive model is the situational model advocated by Malcolm Skilbeck, which emphasises the importance of situation or context in curriculum design. In this model, curriculum designers thoroughly and systematically analyse the situation in which they work for its effect on what they do in the curriculum. The impact of both external and internal factors is assessed and the implications for the curriculum are determined.

Although all steps in the situational model (including situational analysis) need to be completed, they do not need to be followed in any particular order. Curriculum design could begin with a thorough analysis of the situation of the curriculum or the aims, objectives, or outcomes to be achieved, but it could also start from, or be motivated by, a review of content, a revision of assessment, or a thorough consideration of evaluation data. What is possible in curriculum design depends heavily on the context in which the process takes place.

All the elements in curriculum design are linked. They are not separate steps. Content should follow from clear statements of intent and must be derived from considering external and internal context. But equally, content must be delivered by

---

Behavioural objectives*

Acceptable verbs	Unacceptable verbs
● To write	● To know
● To recite	● To understand
● To identify	● To really understand
● To differentiate	● To appreciate
● To solve	● To fully appreciate
● To construct	● To grasp the significance of
● To list	● To enjoy
● To compare	● To believe
● To contrast	● To have faith in

*From Davies I. *Objectives in curriculum design.* London: McGraw Hill, 1976

Clearly stated objectives provide a good starting point, but behavioural objectives are no longer accepted as the "gold standard" in curriculum design

---

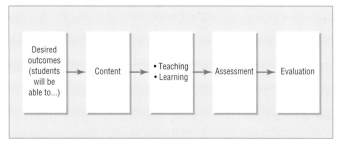

Outcomes based curriculum (defining a curriculum "backwards"—that is, from the starting point of desired outcomes)

Example of statements of intent

Aim
● To produce graduates with knowledge and skills for treating common medical conditions

Objectives
● To identify the mechanisms underlying common diseases of the circulatory system
● To develop skills in history taking for diseases of the circulatory system

Broad outcome
● Graduates will attain knowledge and skills for treating common medical conditions
● Students will identify the mechanisms underlying common diseases of the circulatory system
● Students will acquire skills in history taking for diseases of the circulatory system

---

Situational analysis*

External factors	Internal factors
● Societal expectations and changes	● Students
● Expectations of employers	● Teachers
● Community assumptions and values	● Institutional ethos and structure
● Nature of subject disciplines	● Existing resources
● Nature of support systems	● Problems and shortcomings in existing curriculum
● Expected flow of resources	

*From Reynolds J, Skilbeck M. *Culture and the classroom.* London: Open Books, 1976

appropriate teaching and learning methods and assessed by relevant tools. No one element—for example, assessment—should be decided without considering the other elements.

Curriculum maps

Curriculum maps provide a means of showing the links between the elements of the curriculum. They also display the essential features of the curriculum in a clear and succinct manner. They provide a structure for the systematic organisation of the curriculum, which can be represented diagrammatically and can provide the basis for organising the curriculum into computer databases.

The starting point for the maps may differ depending on the audience. A map for students will place them at the centre and will have a different focus from a map prepared for teachers, administrators, or accrediting authorities. They all have a common purpose, however, in showing the scope, complexity, and cohesion of the curriculum.

Curriculum maps with computer based graphics with "click-on" links are an excellent format. The maps provide one way of tracing the links between the curriculum as planned, as delivered, and as experienced. But like all maps, a balance must be achieved between detail and overall clarity of representation.

Further reading

- Bligh J, Prideaux D, Parsell G. PRISMS: new educational strategies for medical education. *Med Educ* 2001;35:520-1.
- Harden R, Crosby J, Davis M. Outcome based education: part 1—an introduction to outcomes-based education. *Med Teach* 1991;21(1):7-14.
- Harden R. Curriculum mapping: a tool for transparent and authentic teaching and learning. *Med Teach* 2000;23(2):123-7.
- Prideaux D. The emperor's new clothes: from objectives to outcomes. *Med Educ* 2000;34:168-9.
- Print M. *Curriculum development and design.* Sydney: Allen and Unwin, 1993.

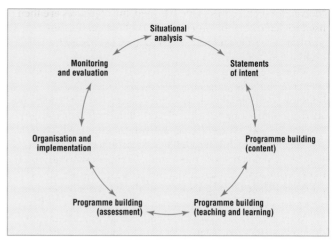

The situational model, which emphasises the importance of situation or context in curriculum design

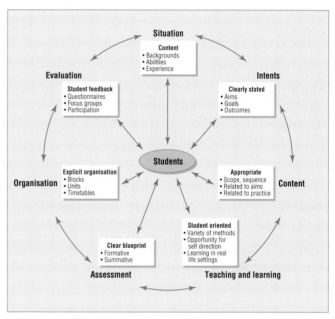

Example of a curriculum map from the students' perspective. Each of the boxes representing the elements of design can be broken down into further units and each new unit can be related to the others to illustrate the interlinking of all the components of the curriculum

3 Problem based learning

Diana Wood

Problem based learning is used in many medical schools in the United Kingdom and worldwide. This article describes this method of learning and teaching in small groups and explains why it has had an important impact on medical education.

What is problem based learning?

In problem based learning (PBL) students use "triggers" from the problem case or scenario to define their own learning objectives. Subsequently they do independent, self directed study before returning to the group to discuss and refine their acquired knowledge. Thus, PBL is not about problem solving per se, but rather it uses appropriate problems to increase knowledge and understanding. The process is clearly defined, and the several variations that exist all follow a similar series of steps.

Group learning facilitates not only the acquisition of knowledge but also several other desirable attributes, such as communication skills, teamwork, problem solving, independent responsibility for learning, sharing information, and respect for others. PBL can therefore be thought of as a small group teaching method that combines the acquisition of knowledge with the development of generic skills and attitudes. Presentation of clinical material as the stimulus for learning enables students to understand the relevance of underlying scientific knowledge and principles in clinical practice.

However, when PBL is introduced into a curriculum, several other issues for curriculum design and implementation need to be tackled. PBL is generally introduced in the context of a defined core curriculum and integration of basic and clinical sciences. It has implications for staffing and learning resources and demands a different approach to timetabling, workload, and assessment. PBL is often used to deliver core material in non-clinical parts of the curriculum. Paper based PBL scenarios form the basis of the core curriculum and ensure that all students are exposed to the same problems. Recently, modified PBL techniques have been introduced into clinical education, with "real" patients being used as the stimulus for learning. Despite the essential ad hoc nature of learning clinical medicine, a "key cases" approach can enable PBL to be used to deliver the core clinical curriculum.

What happens in a PBL tutorial?

PBL tutorials are conducted in several ways. In this article, the examples are modelled on the Maastricht "seven jump" process, but its format of seven steps may be shortened.

A typical PBL tutorial consists of a group of students (usually eight to 10) and a tutor, who facilitates the session. The length of time (number of sessions) that a group stays together with each other and with individual tutors varies between institutions. A group needs to be together long enough to allow good group dynamics to develop but may need to be changed occasionally if personality clashes or other dysfunctional behaviour emerges.

Students elect a chair for each PBL scenario and a "scribe" to record the discussion. The roles are rotated for each scenario. Suitable flip charts or a whiteboard should be used for recording the proceedings. At the start of the session,

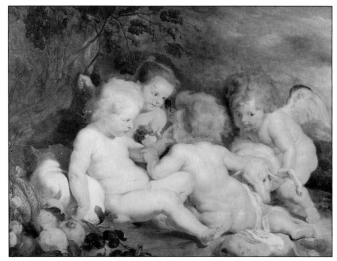

The group learning process: acquiring desirable learning skills

---

Generic skills and attitudes

- Teamwork
- Chairing a group
- Listening
- Recording
- Cooperation
- Respect for colleagues' views
- Critical evaluation of literature
- Self directed learning and use of resources
- Presentation skills

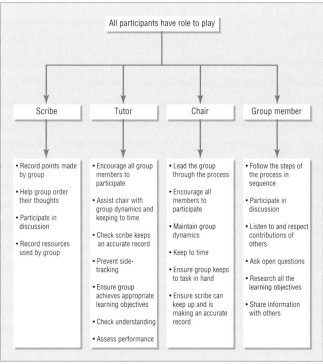

Roles of participants in a PBL tutorial

depending on the trigger material, either the student chair reads out the scenario or all students study the material. If the trigger is a real patient in a ward, clinic, or surgery then a student may be asked to take a clinical history or identify an abnormal physical sign before the group moves to a tutorial room. For each module, students may be given a handbook containing the problem scenarios, and suggested learning resources or learning materials may be handed out at appropriate times as the tutorials progress.

The role of the tutor is to facilitate the proceedings (helping the chair to maintain group dynamics and moving the group through the task) and to ensure that the group achieves appropriate learning objectives in line with those set by the curriculum design team. The tutor may need to take a more active role in step 7 of the process to ensure that all the students have done the appropriate work and to help the chair to suggest a suitable format for group members to use to present the results of their private study. The tutor should encourage students to check their understanding of the material. He or she can do this by encouraging the students to ask open questions and ask each other to explain topics in their own words or by the use of drawings and diagrams.

PBL in curriculum design

PBL may be used either as the mainstay of an entire curriculum or for the delivery of individual courses. In practice, PBL is usually part of an integrated curriculum using a systems based approach, with non-clinical material delivered in the context of clinical practice. A module or short course can be designed to include mixed teaching methods (including PBL) to achieve the learning outcomes in knowledge, skills, and attitudes. A small number of lectures may be desirable to introduce topics or provide an overview of difficult subject material in conjunction with the PBL scenarios. Sufficient time should be allowed each week for students to do the self directed learning required for PBL.

Writing PBL scenarios

PBL is successful only if the scenarios are of high quality. In most undergraduate PBL curriculums the faculty identifies learning objectives in advance. The scenario should lead students to a particular area of study to achieve those learning objectives (see box on page 11).

How to create effective PBL scenarios*

- Learning objectives likely to be defined by the students after studying the scenario should be consistent with the faculty learning objectives
- Problems should be appropriate to the stage of the curriculum and the level of the students' understanding
- Scenarios should have sufficient intrinsic interest for the students or relevance to future practice
- Basic science should be presented in the context of a clinical scenario to encourage integration of knowledge
- Scenarios should contain cues to stimulate discussion and encourage students to seek explanations for the issues presented
- The problem should be sufficiently open, so that discussion is not curtailed too early in the process
- Scenarios should promote participation by the students in seeking information from various learning resources

*Adapted from Dolmans et al. *Med Teacher* 1997;19:185-9

Examples of trigger material for PBL scenarios

- Paper based clinical scenarios
- Experimental or clinical laboratory data
- Photographs
- Video clips
- Newspaper articles
- All or part of an article from a scientific journal
- A real or simulated patient
- A family tree showing an inherited disorder

PBL tutorial process

Step 1—Identify and clarify unfamiliar terms presented in the scenario; scribe lists those that remain unexplained after discussion

Step 2—Define the problem or problems to be discussed; students may have different views on the issues, but all should be considered; scribe records a list of agreed problems

Step 3—"Brainstorming" session to discuss the problem(s), suggesting possible explanations on basis of prior knowledge; students draw on each other's knowledge and identify areas of incomplete knowledge; scribe records all discussion

Step 4—Review steps 2 and 3 and arrange explanations into tentative solutions; scribe organises the explanations and restructures if necessary

Step 5—Formulate learning objectives; group reaches consensus on the learning objectives; tutor ensures learning objectives are focused, achievable, comprehensive, and appropriate

Step 6—Private study (all students gather information related to each learning objective)

Step 7—Group shares results of private study (students identify their learning resources and share their results); tutor checks learning and may assess the group

---

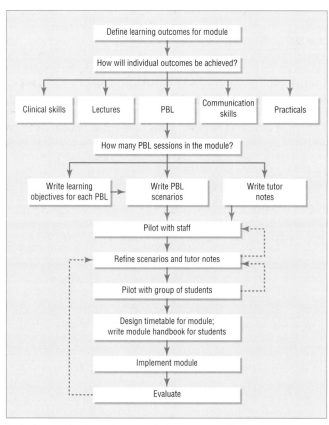

Designing and implementing a curriculum module using PBL supported by other teaching methods

Staff development

Introducing PBL into a course makes new demands on tutors, requiring them to function as facilitators for small group learning rather than acting as providers of information. Staff development is essential and should focus on enabling the PBL tutors to acquire skills in facilitation and in management of group dynamics (including dysfunctional groups).

Tutors should be also given information about the institution's educational strategy and curriculum programme so that they can help students to understand the learning objectives of individual modules in the context of the curriculum as a whole. Methods of assessment and evaluation should be described, and time should be available to discuss anxieties.

Staff may feel uncertain about facilitating a PBL tutorial for a subject in which they do not themselves specialise. Subject specialists may, however, be poor PBL facilitators as they are more likely to interrupt the process and revert to lecturing. None the less, students value expertise, and the best tutors are subject specialists who understand the curriculum and have excellent facilitation skills. However, enthusiastic non-specialist tutors who are trained in facilitation, know the curriculum, and have adequate tutor notes, are good PBL tutors.

Assessment of PBL

Student learning is influenced greatly by the assessment methods used. If assessment methods rely solely on factual recall then PBL is unlikely to succeed in the curriculum. All assessment schedules should follow the basic principles of testing the student in relation to the curriculum outcomes and should use an appropriate range of assessment methods.

Assessment of students' activities in their PBL groups is advisable. Tutors should give feedback or use formative or summative assessment procedures as dictated by the faculty assessment schedule. It is also helpful to consider assessment of the group as a whole. The group should be encouraged to reflect on its PBL performance including its adherence to the process, communication skills, respect for others, and individual contributions. Peer pressure in the group reduces the likelihood of students failing to keep up with workload, and the award of a group mark—added to each individual's assessment schedule—encourages students to achieve the generic goals associated with PBL.

Conclusion

PBL is an effective way of delivering medical education in a coherent, integrated programme and offers several advantages over traditional teaching methods. It is based on principles of adult learning theory, including motivating the students, encouraging them to set their own learning goals, and giving them a role in decisions that affect their own learning.

Predictably, however, PBL does not offer a universal panacea for teaching and learning in medicine, and it has several well recognised disadvantages. Traditional knowledge based assessments of curriculum outcomes have shown little or no difference in students graduating from PBL or traditional curriculums. Importantly, though, students from PBL curriculums seem to have better knowledge retention. PBL also generates a more stimulating and challenging educational environment, and the beneficial effects from the generic attributes acquired through PBL should not be underestimated.

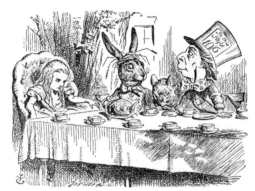

A dysfunctional group: a dominant character may make it difficult for other students to be heard

Advantages and disadvantages of PBL

Advantages of PBL	Disadvantages of PBL
Student centred PBL—It fosters active learning, improved understanding, and retention and development of lifelong learning skills	*Tutors who can't "teach"*—Tutors enjoy passing on their own knowledge and understanding so may find PBL facilitation difficult and frustrating
Generic competencies—PBL allows students to develop generic skills and attitudes desirable in their future practice	*Human resources*—More staff have to take part in the tutoring process
Integration—PBL facilitates an integrated core curriculum	*Other resources*—Large numbers of students need access to the same library and computer resources simultaneously
Motivation—PBL is fun for students and tutors, and the process requires all students to be engaged in the learning process	*Role models*—Students may be deprived access to a particular inspirational teacher who in a traditional curriculum would deliver lectures to a large group
"Deep" learning—PBL fosters deep learning (students interact with learning materials, relate concepts to everyday activities, and improve their understanding)	*Information overload*—Students may be unsure how much self directed study to do and what information is relevant and useful
Constructivist approach—Students activate prior knowledge and build on existing conceptual knowledge frameworks	

Further reading

- Davis MH, Harden RM. AMEE medical education guide number 15: problem-based learning: a practical guide. *Med Teacher* 1999;21:130-40.
- Norman GR, Schmidt HG. Effectiveness of problem-based learning curricula: theory, practice and paper darts. *Med Educ* 2000;34:721-8.
- Albanese M. Problem based learning: why curricula are likely to show little effect on knowledge and clinical skills. *Med Educ* 2000;34:729-38.

Christ and St John with Angels by Peter Paul Rubens is from the collection of the Earl of Pembroke/BAL. The Mad Hatter's Tea Party is by John Tenniel.

PBL scenarios: the importance of linking to faculty learning objectives

PBL scenario 1

A 35 year old part time nurse, presented to her general practitioner, Dr Smith, with a six month history of weight loss (12.7 kg). When questioned, she said she was eating well but had diarrhoea. She also felt exhausted and had developed insomnia. On further questioning she admitted to feeling increasingly hot and shaky and to having muscle weakness in her legs, particularly when climbing stairs. She was normally well and had not seen the doctor since her last pregnancy eight years ago.

A blood test showed the following results:
Free thyroxine 49.7 pmol/l (normal range 11 to 24.5)
Total thyroxine 225 nmol/l (normal range 60 to 150)
Thyroid stimulating hormone < 0.01 mU/l (0.4 to 4.0)

Dr Smith referred her to an endocrinologist at the local hospital where initial investigations confirmed a diagnosis of Graves' disease. She was treated with carbimazole and propranolol for the first month of treatment followed by carbimazole alone. After discussing the therapeutic options, she opted to have iodine-131 treatment.

Faculty learning objectives

- Describe the clinical features of thyrotoxicosis and diagnostic signs of Graves' disease
- Interpret basic thyroid function tests in the light of the pituitary thyroid axis and feedback mechanisms
- List the types of treatment for thyrotoxicosis including their indications, mode of action, and potential side effects

Notes

This scenario is part of a core endocrinology and metabolism module for third year undergraduate medical students. The faculty learning objectives relate to the scenario; the problem is relevant to the level of study and integrates basic science with clinical medicine. The combination of basic science, clinical medicine, and therapeutics should lead to extensive discussion and broadly based self directed learning

PBL scenario 2

Mr JB, a 58 year old car mechanic with a history of chronic obstructive pulmonary disease, was at work when he complained of pain in his chest. The pain steadily got worse and he described an aching in his jaw and left arm. One hour after the pain started he collapsed and his colleagues called an ambulance. When he arrived at the local accident and emergency department, Mr JB was pale, sweaty, and in severe pain.

Examination showed:
Blood pressure 80/60 mm Hg
Heart rate 64 beats/min
Electrocardiography showed anterolateral myocardial infarction

He was treated with diamorphine, metoclopramide, and aspirin. As the accident and emergency staff were preparing to give him streptokinase, he had a cardiac arrest. Electrocardiography showed asystolic cardiac arrest. Despite all efforts, resuscitation failed.

Faculty learning objectives

- List the risk factors for myocardial infarction
- Describe a rehabilitation programme for patients who have had a myocardial infarction

Notes

This scenario is part of a core module in the cardiorespiratory system for first year undergraduate medical students. The scenario is complex for students with limited clinical experience. The faculty learning objectives relate to public health and epidemiological aspects of ischaemic heart disease. For increased impact, the faculty illustrated the case with a dramatic scenario. Students would be unlikely to arrive at the same objectives, probably concentrating on clinical aspects of acute myocardial infarction and its management

4 Evaluation

Jill Morrison

Evaluation is an essential part of the educational process. The focus of evaluation is on local quality improvement and is analogous to clinical audit. Medical schools require evaluation as part of their quality assurance procedures, but the value of evaluation is much greater than the provision of simple audit information. It provides evidence of how well students' learning objectives are being achieved and whether teaching standards are being maintained. Importantly, it also enables the curriculum to evolve. A medical curriculum should constantly develop in response to the needs of students, institutions, and society. Evaluation can check that the curriculum is evolving in the desired way. It should be viewed positively as contributing to the academic development of an institution and its members.

Evaluation versus research

Evaluation and educational research are similar activities but with important differences. Research is usually aimed at producing generalisable results that can be published in peer reviewed literature, and it requires ethical and other safeguards. Evaluation is generally carried out for local use and does not usually require ethics committee approval. Evaluation has to be carefully considered by curriculum committees, however, to ensure that it is being carried out ethically. Finally, evaluation is a continuous process, whereas research may not become continuous if the answer to the question is found.

What should be evaluated

Evaluation may cover the process and/or outcome of any aspect of education, including the delivery and content of teaching. Questions about delivery may relate to organisation—for example, administrative arrangements, physical environment, and teaching methods. Information may also be sought about the aptitude of the teacher(s) involved. The content may be evaluated for its level (it should not be too easy or too difficult), its relevance to curriculum objectives, and integration with previous learning.

Outcome measures may show the impact of the curriculum on the knowledge, skills, attitudes, and behaviour of students. Kirkpatrick described four levels on which to focus evaluation; these have recently been adapted for use in health education evaluation by Barr and colleagues. Some indication of these attributes may be obtained by specific methods of inquiry—for example, by analysing data from student assessments.

Evaluation in curriculum planning

Evaluation should be designed at the start of developing a curriculum, not added as an afterthought. When an educational need has been identified, the first stage is to define the learning outcomes for the curriculum. The goals of the evaluation should be clearly articulated and linked to the outcomes.

Clarifying the goals of evaluation will help to specify the evidence needed to determine success or failure of the training. .A protocol should then be prepared so that individual responsibilities are clearly outlined.

Purpose of evaluation

- To ensure teaching is meeting students' learning needs
- To identify areas where teaching can be improved
- To inform the allocation of faculty resources
- To provide feedback and encouragement for teachers
- To support applications for promotion by teachers
- To identify and articulate what is valued by medical schools
- To facilitate development of the curriculum

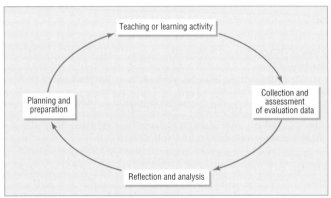

Evaluation cycle. From Wilkes et al (see "Further reading" box)

Kirkpatrick's four levels on which to focus evaluation*

- Level 1—Learner's reactions
- Level 2a—Modification of attitudes and perceptions
- Level 2b—Acquisition of knowledge and skills
- Level 3—Change in behaviour
- Level 4a—Change in organisational practice
- Level 4b—Benefits to patients or clients

*Adapted by Barr et al (see "Further reading" box)

The full impact of the curriculum may not be known until some time after the student has graduated

---

Questions to ask when planning an evaluation

- What are the goals of the evaluation?
- From whom and in what form will data be collected?
- Who will collect and analyse data?
- What type of analysis, interpretation, and decision rules will be used and by whom?
- Who will see the results of the evaluation?

Designing evaluation

An ideal evaluation method would be reliable, valid, acceptable, and inexpensive. Unfortunately, ideal methods for evaluating teaching in medical schools are scarce.

Establishing the reliability and validity of instruments and methods of evaluation can take many years and be costly. Testing and retesting of instruments to establish their psychometric properties without any additional benefit for students or teachers is unlikely to be popular with them. There is a need for robust "off the shelf" instruments that can be used to evaluate curriculums reliably. The process of evaluation itself may produce a positive educational impact if it emphasises those elements that are considered valuable and important by medical schools.

Participation by students

Several issues should be considered before designing an evaluation that collects information from students.

Competence—Students can be a reliable and valid source of information. They are uniquely aware of what they can consume, and they observe teaching daily. They are also an inexpensive resource. Daily contact, however, does not mean that students are skilled in evaluation. Evaluation by students should be limited to areas in which they are competent to judge.

Ownership—Students who are not committed to an evaluation may provide poor information. They need to feel ownership for an evaluation by participating in its development. The importance of obtaining the information and the type of information needed must be explicit. Usually the results of an evaluation will affect only subsequent cohorts of students, so current students must be convinced of the value of providing data.

Sampling—Students need to feel that their time is respected. If they are asked to fill out endless forms they will resent the waste of their time. If they become bored by tedious repetition, the reliability of the data will deteriorate. One solution is to use different sampling strategies for evaluating different elements of a curriculum. If reliable information can be obtained from 100 students, why collect data from 300?

Anonymity is commonly advocated as a guard against bias when information is collected from students. However, those who support asking students to sign evaluation forms say that this helps to create a climate of responsible peer review. If students are identifiable from the information they provide, this must not affect their progress. Data should be collected centrally and students' names removed so that they cannot be identified by teachers whom they have criticised.

Feedback—Students need to know that their opinions are valued, so they should be told of the results of the evaluation and given details of the resulting action.

Methods of evaluation

Evaluation may involve subjective and objective measures and qualitative and quantitative approaches. The resources devoted to evaluation should reflect its importance, but excessive data collection should be avoided. A good system should be easy to administer and use information that is readily available.

Interviews—Individual interviews with students are useful if the information is sensitive—for example, when a teacher has received poor ratings from students, and the reasons are not clear. A group interview can provide detailed views from students or teachers. A teaching session can end with reflection by the group.

Characteristics of an ideal evaluation

- Reliability
- Validity
- Acceptability—to evaluator and to person being evaluated
- Inexpensiveness

To reduce possible bias in evaluation, collect views from more than one group of people—for example, students, teachers, other clinicians, and patients

---

Areas of competence of students to evaluate teaching and curriculum

- Design: whether the curriculum enables students to reach their learning objectives; whether it fits well with other parts of the curriculum
- Delivery: attributes of teacher and methods used
- Administrative arrangements

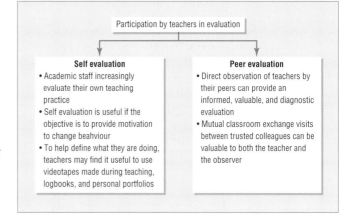

Issues relating to students' participation in evaluation may also apply to teachers, but self evaluation and peer evaluation are also relevant

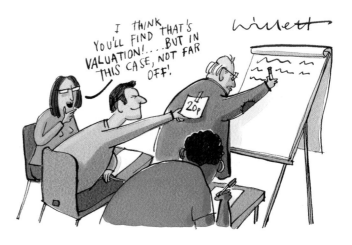

Surveys—Questionnaires are useful for obtaining information from large numbers of students or teachers about the teaching process. Electronic methods for administering questionnaires may improve response rates. The quality of the data, however, is only as good as the questions asked, and the data may not provide the reasons for a poorly rated session.

Information from student assessment—Data from assessment are useful for finding out if students have achieved the learning outcomes of a curriculum. A downward trend in examination results over several cohorts of students may indicate a deficiency in the curriculum. Caution is needed when interpreting this source of information, as students' examination performance depends as much on their application, ability, and motivation as on the teaching.

Completing the evaluation cycle

The main purpose of evaluation is to inform curriculum development. No curriculum is perfect in design and delivery. If the results of an evaluation show that no further development is needed, doubt is cast on the methods of evaluation or the interpretation of the results.

This does not mean that curriculums should be in a constant state of change, but that the results of evaluation to correct deficiencies are acted on, that methods continue to improve, and that content is updated. Then the process starts all over again.

Worked example

Background
Clinical teaching staff think that students are becoming weaker at examining cranial nerves. The examination scores for that part of the objective structured clinical examination (OSCE) carried out at the end of year three show a decline over several years. Three focus groups are held with students in year four, and several clinical teachers are interviewed. The results suggest that the decline is due to fewer appropriate patients presenting at outpatient sessions where cranial nerve examination is taught and to a lack of opportunities for practising examination skills.

Intervention
A teaching session is designed for delivery in the clinical skills centre. After that, students should be able to do a systematic examination of cranial nerves. They should also recognise normal signs and know which common abnormalities to look for. Sessions are timetabled for practising skills learnt during the teaching session.

Evaluation
A questionnaire is developed for completion by a third of students. It seeks their views on the teaching process, including the teaching skills of the tutor, physical aspects of the teaching environment, appropriateness of the teaching material, and opportunities for practising examination skills. Outcome measures include comparison of examination scores for students in the previous cohort with those participating in the teaching session, plus a questionnaire for all clinical supervisors for neurology in the following year to get their views about students' examination skills. A tenth of students with a range of scores in the relevant part of the OSCE are interviewed to find out the reasons for their varied scores. The evaluation results are disseminated widely to staff and students.

> Questionnaire surveys are the most common evaluation tool

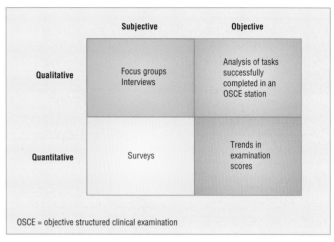

OSCE = objective structured clinical examination

Examples of methods of evaluation

Key points

Evaluation should:
- Enable strategic development of a curriculum
- Be a positive process that contributes to the academic development of a medical school

The goals of an evaluation should:
- Be clearly articulated
- Be linked to the outcomes of the teaching

When carrying out an evaluation:
- More than one source and type of information should be sought
- The results should be fed back to participants and details of the resulting action given

Learners need:
- To be involved in developing an evaluation
- To feel their time is respected
- To know their opinions are valued and acted on

Evaluators must:
- Act on the results of the evaluation to correct deficiencies, improve methods, and update content
- Repeat the process

Further reading
- Robson C. *Small scale evaluation*. London: Sage, 2000.
- Cohen L, Manion L. *Research methods in education*. 4th ed. London: Routledge, 1994.
- Snell L, Tallett S, Haist S, Hays R, Norcini J, Prince K, et al. A review of the evaluation of clinical teaching: new perspectives and challenges. *Med Educ* 2000;34:862-70.
- Barr H, Freeth D, Hammick M, Koppel, Reeves S. *Evaluations of interprofessional education: a United Kingdom review of health and social care*. London: CAIPE/BERA, 2000.
- Wilkes M, Bligh J. Evaluating educational interventions. *BMJ* 1999;318:1269-72.

5 Teaching large groups

Peter Cantillon

Lecturing or large group teaching is one of the oldest forms of teaching. Whatever their reputation, lectures are an efficient means of transferring knowledge and concepts to large groups. They can be used to stimulate interest, explain concepts, provide core knowledge, and direct student learning.

However, they should not be regarded as an effective way of teaching skills, changing attitudes, or encouraging higher order thinking. Large group formats tend to encourage passive learning. Students receive information but have little opportunity to process or critically appraise the new knowledge offered.

How can lectures be used to maximise learning and provide opportunities for student interaction? This article will supply some of the answers and should help you to deliver better, more interactive lectures.

Getting your bearings

It is important to find out as much as possible about the context of the lecture—that is, where it fits into the course of which it is part.

An understanding of the context will allow you to prepare a lecture that is both appropriate and designed to move students on from where they are.

Helping students to learn in lectures

An important question for any lecturer to consider when planning a teaching session is, "how can I help my students to learn during my lecture?" There are several different techniques you can use to aid student learning in a large group setting.

Helping your students to learn

- Use concrete examples to illustrate abstract principles
- Give handouts of the lecture slides, with space to write notes
- Give handouts with partially completed diagrams and lists for the students to complete during or after the lecture
- Allow for pauses in the delivery to give students time to write notes
- Check for understanding by asking questions or by running a mini quiz

---

Planning your lecture

It is important to distinguish between the knowledge and concepts that are essential (need to know) and those which, though interesting, are not part of the core message (nice to know).

The aims of the lecture should be clearly defined ("what do I hope to achieve with this lecture?"). These will help to define the teaching methods and the structure. If, for example, the purpose of the lecture is to introduce new knowledge and concepts, then a classic lecture structure might be most appropriate.

On the other hand, if the purpose is to make the students aware of different approaches to a particular clinical problem, a problem oriented design in which alternative approaches are presented and discussed might be a more appropriate format.

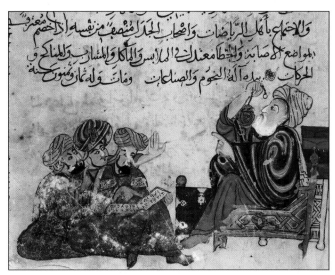

A lecturer holds forth …

What you need to know before planning a lecture

- How your lecture fits into the students' course or curriculum
- The students' knowledge of your subject—try to get a copy of the lecture and tutorial list for the course
- How the course (and your lecture) will be assessed
- The teaching methods that the students are accustomed to

> **The successful teacher is no longer on a height, pumping knowledge at high pressure into passive receptacles … he is a senior student anxious to help his juniors.**
>
> **William Osler (1849-1919)**

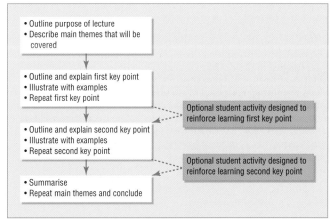

- Outline purpose of lecture
- Describe main themes that will be covered

- Outline and explain first key point
- Illustrate with examples
- Repeat first key point

  ⟶ Optional student activity designed to reinforce learning first key point

- Outline and explain second key point
- Illustrate with examples
- Repeat second key point

  ⟶ Optional student activity designed to reinforce learning second key point

- Summarise
- Repeat main themes and conclude

Example of a lecture plan with a classic structure

Choosing teaching media

When you have selected the content of the lecture and placed it into a working structure, the next consideration is how to deliver the message. Which teaching media should be used (for example, slides, overheads, handouts, quizzes)? The most appropriate media will differ depending on the venue, class size, and topic.

Choosing the medium for delivering the lecture

- Which teaching media are available at the teaching venue?
- Which teaching media are you familiar with? (It is not always appropriate to experiment with new media)
- Which medium will best illustrate the concepts and themes that you want to teach the students?
- Which medium would encourage students to learn through interaction during your lecture?

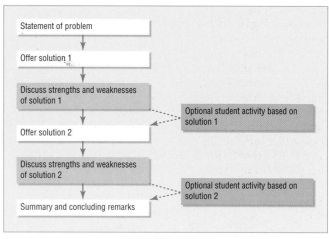

Example of a lecture plan with a problem oriented structure

Getting started

In the first moments of a lecture it is important that the students are given some sense of place and direction. Thus a brief summary of the previous lecture and an indication of the major themes and learning objectives for the current session provide both you and the students with a relatively easy start. If you are working with a new group it may be useful to indicate the ground rules for the session—for example, "switch off mobile phones," or "ask questions at any time."

Encouraging students to interact

Students learn well by "doing." Yet there is an understandable tendency for students to regard lectures as an opportunity to sit back, be entertained, and "soak up" the learning. However, you can use various methods to encourage students to take a more active part in the learning process.

Students' attention (and recall) is best at the beginning and end of a lecture. Recall can be improved by changing the format of your lecture part way through. It is also important when planning a lecture to think about activities and exercises that will break up the presentation.

Ask questions

It is useful to ask questions of the group at various stages in the lecture, to check comprehension and promote discussion. Many lecturers are intimidated by the silence following a question and fall into the trap of answering it themselves. Wait for the answers to come. It takes time for students to move from listening to thinking mode. A simple tip is to count slowly to 10 in your head—a question is almost certain to arrive.

Get students to ask you questions

An alternative to getting students to answer questions is to ask them to direct questions at you. A good way of overcoming students' normal fear of embarrassment is to ask them to prepare questions in groups of two or three. Questions can then be invited from groups at random. When asked a question, you should repeat it out loud to ensure that the whole group is aware of what was asked. Seeking answers to the question from other students, before adding your own views, can increase the level of interaction further.

Handouts

- Handouts can encourage better learning if they allow students more time to listen and think
- Handouts should provide a scaffold on which students can build their understanding of a topic
- Handouts should provide a summary of the major themes while avoiding an exhaustive explanation of each
- Handouts can be used to direct further learning, by including exercises and questions with suggested reading lists

---

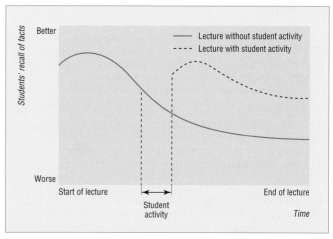

Graph showing effect of students' interaction on their ability to recall what they have heard in a lecture. Adapted from Bligh, 2000 (see "Recommended reading" box)

"Tell me, and I forget. Show me, and I remember. Involve me, and I understand"

Chinese proverb

Brainstorming

Brainstorming is a technique for activating the students' knowledge or current understanding of an issue or theme. The lecturer invites answers to a question or problem from the audience and writes them, without comment, on a board or overhead. After a short period, usually about two or three minutes, the lecturer reviews the list of "answers" with the class. The answers can be used to provide material for the next part of the lecture or to give students an idea of where they are before they move on. By writing answers in a way that can be seen by everyone in the audience, you allow the students to learn from each other.

Buzz groups

Buzz groups also encourage interaction. They consist of groups of two to five students working for a few minutes on a question, problem, or exercise set by the lecturer. Buzz group activity is a useful means of getting students to process and use new information to solve problems. At the end of the buzz group session, the teacher can either continue with the lecture or check the results of the exercise by asking one or two groups to present their views. Remember that in an amphitheatre lecture hall, students can sit on their own desks to interact with the students behind them.

Mini-assessments

Mini-assessments and exercises are used in lectures to help students to recognise gaps in their learning and to encourage them to use new material in practice. Brief assessments can also allow the lecturer to measure how well the messages are being understood. Students could be asked, for example, to complete a brief, multiple choice questionnaire or a "one-minute" paper. The timing of quizzes and exercises will depend on what is required. An assessment of prior learning would be best at the start of a lecture, whereas an estimate of learning from the current session might be best carried out towards the end of the lecture.

How to end your lecture

At the end of a lecture it is important to summarise the key points and direct students toward further learning. You may present the key points on a slide or overhead. Alternatively, you may go through the main headings on a handout. Students are encouraged to learn more about a subject if they are set tasks or exercises that will require them to look further than the lecture notes for answers and ideas. The end of a lecture is also a common time for questions. Students may find the use of a one-minute paper a useful tool to help them to identify concepts and impressions that need clarification.

Evaluating your lecture

Practice does make perfect, but the process of developing as a lecturer is greatly helped if some effort is made to evaluate performance. Evaluation involves answering questions such as "how did I do?" or "what did the students learn?"

A lecture can be evaluated in different ways. If the students are to be used as a source of feedback, the following methods are useful:
- Ask a sample of the students if you can read their lecture notes—this exercise gives some insight into what students have learned and understood
- Ask for verbal feedback from individual students
- Ask the students to complete a one-minute paper

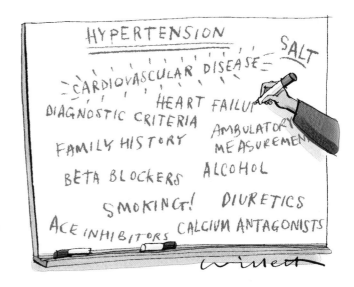

"One-minute" paper worksheet

Name: _____

Date: _____

Lecture title: _____

Directions: Take a moment to think about the lecture you have just attended, and then answer the following questions.

1. What was the most important thing you learned in today's lecture?

_____

2. What question remains uppermost in your mind at the end of today's lecture?

_____

3. What was the "muddiest point" in today's lecture?

_____

Example of a one-minute paper

Please rate the lecture on the following items

	Strongly agree	Slightly agree	Slightly disagree	Strongly disagree
Clear				
Interesting				
Easy to take notes from				
Well organised				
Relevant to the course				

Example of an evaluation form focusing on the lecture. Adapted from Brown et al, 2001 (see "Recommended reading" box)

- Ask the students to complete an evaluation questionnaire.

If you want to evaluate your teaching style and delivery, peers can be a useful source of feedback:

- Ask a colleague to observe part or all of a lecture and provide feedback afterwards. It is important to inform the observer what aspects of the lecturing process you want evaluated—for example, clarity, logical flow, effectiveness of the media used
- Videotape the lecture for private viewing, and arrange a joint viewing with a colleague later.

Lectures are still a common teaching method in both undergraduate and postgraduate medical education. Their continued popularity is due to the fact that they represent an effective and efficient means of teaching new concepts and knowledge. This article has emphasised the importance of good lecture planning and of the inclusion of student interaction to ensure effective learning.

Recommended reading

- Newble DI, Cannon R. *A handbook for medical teachers.* 4th ed. Dordrecht, Netherlands: Kluwer Academic, 2001.
- Gibbs G, Habeshaw T. *Preparing to teach.* Bristol: Technical and Educational Services, 1989.
- Bligh DA. *What's the use of lectures?* San Francisco: Jossey-Bass, 2000.
- Brown G, Manogue M. AMEE medical education guide No 22: refreshing lecturing: a guide for lecturers. *Medical Teacher* 2001;23:231-44.

Please rate the lecturer on the following items

	Strongly agree	Slightly agree	Slightly disagree	Strongly disagree
Was enthusiastic				
Was clearly audible				
Seemed confident				
Gave clear explanations				
Encouraged participation				

Example of an evaluation form focusing on the lecturer rather than the lecture. Adapted from Brown et al, 2001 (see "Recommended reading" box)

6 Teaching small groups

David Jaques

Group discussion plays a valuable role in the all-round education of students, whether in problem based learning and team projects or in the more traditional academic scenario of the tutorial or seminar. When it works well, discussion can allow students to negotiate meanings, express themselves in the language of the subject, and establish closer contact with academic staff than more formal methods permit. Discussion can also develop the more instrumental skills of listening, presenting ideas, persuading, and working as part of a team. But perhaps most importantly, discussion in small groups can or should give students the chance to monitor their own learning and thus gain a degree of self direction and independence in their studies.

All these worthy aims require active participation and the ready expression of ideas. Yet it frequently doesn't work out this way. Indeed many tutors too readily fall back on their reserve positions of authority, expert, and prime talker. Many of the problems associated with leading small groups effectively are likely to be exacerbated with larger groups. So how can we avoid the common traps?

If you are leading a group discussion you will need to consider both the configuration of the group and your own behaviour. Groups often communicate poorly because the physical conditions make it difficult to communicate. For example, in a group of 10 students seated round a rectangular table, at least four students on either side of the table have no eye contact with each other, thus reducing participation. If you ask and answer questions all the time, even less interaction is likely.

If a group sits in a circle without a table, communication is likely to be easier. When the discussion has started, it is your responsibility as discussion leader to listen to and respond to the whole group. Listening becomes a problem when the students regard you as an expert or you engage with one or two of the more vocal students rather than the whole group.

More structure, less intervention

Being a democratic discussion leader involves making the right sort of nudges and interventions. The role can be made a lot less demanding by using more structure and less intervention in the group process. The rest of this article shows how clear and purposeful group structures can help to bypass many of the problems outlined above, by delegating responsibility for group interaction (and therefore for learning) to the students.

Group structures and processes

You can minimise your internal involvement in the group process by organising or structuring groups into smaller units, especially when the group process is likely to be problematical. This is particularly so when you wish to mobilise a sense of coherence and full participation among a largish group of students. A sequence of tasks might then be set. For example:
- Students work individually for five minutes drawing up a list
- They share their ideas in pairs for 10 minutes
- In groups of four to six, students write up categories on a large sheet of paper
- This is followed by 25 minutes of open discussion among the groups.

> **"By separating teaching from learning, we have teachers who do not listen and students who do not talk"**
> **Based on Palmer P (*The Courage to Teach.* Jossey Bass, 1998)**

Problems associated with leading effective small groups
- The teacher gives a lecture rather than conducting a dialogue
- The teacher talks too much
- Students cannot be encouraged to talk except with difficulty; they will not talk to each other, but will only respond to questions from the tutor
- Students do not prepare for the sessions
- One student dominates or blocks the discussion
- The students want to be given the solutions to problems rather than discuss them

---

> **Your own behaviour can have an enormous effect on how the group functions**

Techniques for effective facilitation in group discussion
- Ensure that group members have an agreed set of ground rules—for example, not talking at the same time as another group member
- Ensure that the students are clear about the tasks to be carried out
- When you present a question don't answer it yourself or try to reformulate it—count to 10 silently before speaking again
- When you have something you *could* say (which could be most of the time), count to 10 again
- Look round the group both when you are speaking and when a student is speaking. That way the students will quickly recognise that they are addressing the group rather than just you. It will allow you to pick up cues from those who want to speak but are either a bit slow or inhibited

---

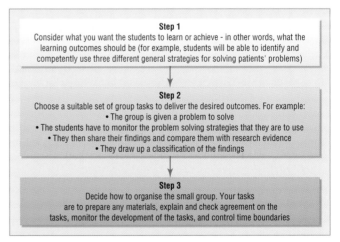

Step 1
Consider what you want the students to learn or achieve - in other words, what the learning outcomes should be (for example, students will be able to identify and competently use three different general strategies for solving patients' problems)

Step 2
Choose a suitable set of group tasks to deliver the desired outcomes. For example:
- The group is given a problem to solve
- The students have to monitor the problem solving strategies that they are to use
- They then share their findings and compare them with research evidence
- They draw up a classification of the findings

Step 3
Decide how to organise the small group. Your tasks are to prepare any materials, explain and check agreement on the tasks, monitor the development of the tasks, and control time boundaries

Planning the structure of a small discussion group

Your role in this kind of situation may be to move round checking that everyone understands and accepts the task and is doing it in an appropriate way and to encourage completion as the end point approaches. You could leave the room for a while and let the groups work without supervision.

The following group structures require some assertive leadership to set up but allow you to take a back seat as the process itself takes over the direction of events.

Group round

Each person has a brief time—say, 20 seconds or one minute—to say something in turn round the group. The direction round the group can be decided by the first contributor, or members can speak in a random order. More interest and energy is usually generated, however, if the first person chooses who should go second, the second who should go third, and so on.

Buzz groups

With larger groups a break is often needed:
- To provide a stimulating change in the locus of attention
- For you to gain some idea of what the students know
- For the students to check their own understanding.

During a discussion students could be asked to turn to their neighbour to discuss for a few minutes any difficulties in understanding, to answer a prepared question, or to speculate on what they think will happen next in the proceedings. This will bring a sense of participation and some lively feedback. Buzz groups enable students to express difficulties they would have been unwilling to reveal to the whole class. (A variation is to allocate three or five minutes each way to the pairs—each phase is for one-way communication.)

Snowball groups

Snowball groups (or pyramids) are an extension of buzz groups. Pairs join up to form fours, then fours to eights. These groups of eight report back to the whole group. This developing pattern of group interaction can ensure comprehensive participation, especially when it starts with individuals writing down their ideas before sharing them. To avoid students becoming bored with repeated discussion of the same points, it is a good idea to use increasingly sophisticated tasks as the groups gets larger.

Fishbowls

The usual fishbowl configuration has an inner group discussing an issue or topic while the outer group listens, looking for themes, patterns, or soundness of argument or uses a group behaviour checklist to give feedback to the group on its functioning. The roles may then be reversed.

Crossover groups

Students are divided into subgroups that are subsequently split up to form new groups in such a way as to maximise the crossing over of information. A colour or number coding in the first groupings enables a simple relocation—from, for example, three groups of four students to four groups of three, with each group in the second configuration having one from each of the first.

Circular questioning

In circular questioning each member of the group asks a question in turn. In its simplest version, one group member formulates a question relevant to the theme or problem and puts it to the person opposite, who has a specified time (say, one

> To encourage group interaction consider breaking a larger group into smaller groups of five or six students; organise membership on a heterogeneous or random basis to prevent cliques forming

> Group rounds are particularly useful at the beginning of any meeting so that everyone is involved from the start and, depending on what the group is asked to speak about, as a way of checking on learning issues

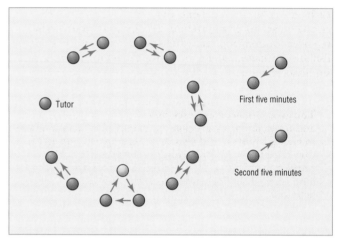

Buzz groups, with pairs for one-way, five-minute communication

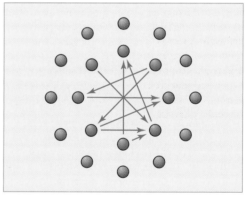

Fishbowl structure—inside group discusses, outside group listens in

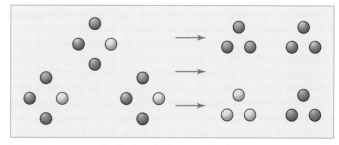

Crossover groups—redistribution of 12 students (each allocated one of four colours) for second period of session

or two minutes) to answer it. Follow up questions can be asked if time permits. The questioning and answering continues clockwise round the group until everyone has contributed, at which time a review of questions and answers can take place. This could also include answers that others would like to have given. Alternatively, you or the students could prepare the questions on cards. You could also mix the best of the students' questions with some of your own.

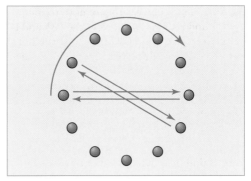

Circular questioning

Horseshoe groups

This method allows you to alternate between the lecture and discussion formats, a common practice in workshops. Groups are arranged around tables, with each group in a horseshoe formation with the open end facing the front. You can thus talk formally from the board for a time before switching to presenting a group task. Subsequent reporting from each group can induce boredom. To avoid this danger, the tutor can circulate written reports for comment; get groups to interview each other publicly or get one member of each group to circulate; ask groups to produce and display posters; ask the reporters from each group to form an inner group in a fishbowl formation; or use the crossover method to move students around.

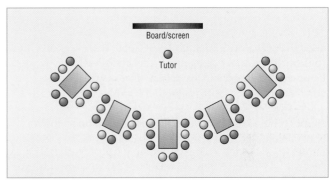

Horseshoe groups

> **The group structures described require an explicit task and topic, and they are possible only if the furniture is movable. Tutors could also consider experimenting with furniture to see if other group structures work. The physical configuration is a strong determinant of social (and hence learning) processes, as is the sequence of activities**

Conclusion

This article has emphasised the choices available to you in working with groups. Some of these involve more skilled and sensitive handling of group process from within the group; others require imaginative management in the setting of tasks and the organising of purposeful activities for subgroups. Well organised and purposeful group discussion can create a firm foundation for qualities such as openness, networking, and proactive communication—important ingredients in the process of personal and organisational change. The value of effective group management in professional development and lifelong learning cannot be underestimated.

Recommended reading

- Brookfield S, Preskill S. *Discussion as a way of teaching—tools and techniques for university teachers.* Buckingham: Open University Press, 1999.
- Forster F, Hounsell D, Thompson S. *Tutoring and demonstrating—a handbook.* Sheffield: Universities' and Colleges' Staff Development Agency, 1995.
- Habeshaw T, Habeshaw S, Gibbs G. *53 interesting things to do in your seminars and tutorials.* Bristol: Technical and Educational Services, 1992.
- Jaques D. *Learning in groups.* 3rd ed. London: Kogan Page, 2000.
- Tiberius R. *Small group teaching: a trouble-shooting guide.* London: Kogan Page, 1999.

7 One to one teaching and feedback

Jill Gordon

> "My method (is) to lead my students by hand to the practice of medicine, taking them every day to see patients in the public hospital, that they may hear the patients' symptoms and see their physical findings. Then I question the students as to what they have noted in the patients and about their thoughts and perceptions regarding the cause of the illness and the principles of treatment"
>
> **Dr Franciscus de la Boe Sylvius, 17th century professor of medicine at the University of Leyden, Netherlands**

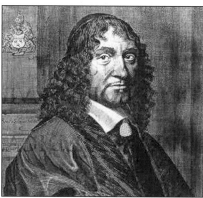

Dr Franciscus de la Boe Sylvius

Although it is not clear whether Dr Sylvius (above) was describing his teaching method in relation to a group of students or to a succession of individual students, he understood the essential features of clinical education. He understood, for example, the need for active learning in an authentic clinical setting.

Dr Sylvius also understood another important feature of one to one teaching—close behavioural observation (of each other, teacher and learner). No other setting provides the same opportunity for this. Dr Sylvius led his students "by [the] hand." He cared about his role as a teacher. In the closely observed one to one relationship your unguarded statements, your reactions under pressure, and your opinions about other people and the world at large are all magnified.

Just as you cannot hide from the learner, so the learner's knowledge, skills, and attitudes will become apparent to you. Provided that you have created a trusting relationship, you can discuss his or her personal and professional attitudes and values in a way that is seldom possible in a larger group. This is perhaps one of the key benefits of one to one teaching.

Another feature of one to one teaching is the opportunity to adjust what you teach to the learner's needs—"customise" your teaching. In 1978 Ausubel and colleagues suggested that the secret of education is to find out what the learner already knows and teach accordingly. In a lecture, tutorial, or seminar you cannot hope to diagnose and respond to every individual's learning needs, but a one to one relationship provides an opportunity to match the learning experience to the learner.

One to one teaching is perhaps one of the most powerful ways of "influencing students." You can create opportunities for active learning in authentic clinical settings while modelling desirable personal and professional attributes.

Stott and Davis in 1979 promoted the idea that one to one primary care consultations offer exceptional but often unrealised potential. The principles used in primary care consultations can be applied to one to one teaching, and the secret is forethought and planning.

Wards, operating theatres, general practice, and community clinics provide a context for active learning

---

As a teacher, you are an important role model whether you wish it or not

---

What's different about one to one teaching?

	Lecture	Seminar	PBL group	Clinical tutorial	One to one clinical attachment
Efficiency*	High	Medium	Low	Low	Very low
Active learning	Low (usually)	Variable	High	Medium to high	Very high
Mutual feedback	Low	Medium	High	Medium to high	Very high
Modelling behaviour in real life setting	Low	Low	Medium	High	Very high

PBL = problem based learning.
*Based on student numbers.

Plan ahead—ask yourself some important questions

- What is the main purpose of the one to one attachment?
- Do you know why it is part of the learning programme?
- What are the learner's needs?
- How will you gauge how effectively you have met the learner's needs?
- How would you like this learner to describe the experience to a peer?

Exceptional potential of one to one teaching

- It tackles current learning needs
- It promotes autonomy and self directed learning
- It links prior knowledge with new clinical experiences
- It enables opportunistic teaching

Provide an orientation

Most of us recall clinical teachers whose social skills amounted to a brief glance and a grunt. Times have changed, or should have. Find out and remember the learner's name—a simple but important courtesy. Outline the special opportunities and benefits that the attachment can provide. Ask the learner to prepare a learning plan and then compare the learner's plan to your own expectations. Once the plan has been agreed, don't shelve it—refer to it during the attachment and modify as necessary.

Agree on the ground rules

Ground rules are both practical (punctuality, dress, access to patient records) and philosophical (respect for patients and colleagues, confidentiality, consent, openness to different points of view). If these have been spelled out on day 1, you won't be caught out later. Make sure that the learner knows how much time you will be able to spend in observing, teaching, and giving feedback and what you expect in return.

Ask helpful questions

Open ended questions are generally better than closed questions at the beginning of the exchange. A small number of closed questions later in the conversation help you to "diagnose" just how much the learner knows and understands. Avoid questions that require nothing but recall. Try to formulate questions that assume an appropriate amount of knowledge, but build in higher order thinking and/or higher order skills. You might ask the learner, for example, to explain to you (as if you were the patient) the mechanisms behind a condition such as asthma or hypertension. This simulates clinical interface with a patient—testing recall, understanding, and communications skills all at once.

Give feedback

Learners value feedback highly, and valid feedback is based on observation. Deal with observable behaviours and be practical, timely, and concrete. The one to one relationship enables you to give feedback with sensitivity and in private. Begin by asking the learner to tell you what he or she feels confident of having done well and what he or she would like to improve. Follow up with your own observations of what was done well (be specific), and then outline one or two points that could help the student to improve.

Encourage reflection

Just as many learning opportunities are wasted if they are not accompanied by feedback from an observer, so too are they wasted if the learner cannot reflect honestly on his or her performance. One to one teaching is ideally suited to encouraging reflective practice, because you can model the way a reflective practitioner behaves. Two key skills are (a) "unpacking" your clinical reasoning and decision making processes and (b) describing and discussing the ethical values and beliefs that guide you in patient care.

Use other one to one teachers

Senior medical students, junior doctors, registrars, nurses, and allied health professionals are all potential teachers. When

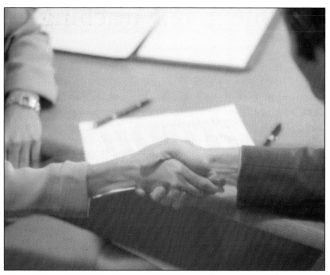

Find out and remember the learner's name—a simple but important courtesy

> **Skilful teaching is not unlike skilful history taking**

> "If musicians learned to play their instruments as physicians learn to interview patients, the procedure would consist of presenting in lectures or maybe in a demonstration or two the theory and mechanisms of the music-producing ability of the instrument and telling him to produce a melody. The instructor of course, would not be present to observe or listen to the student's efforts, but would be satisfied with the student's subsequent verbal report of what came out of the instrument."
>
> George Engel, after visiting 70 medical schools in North America

Monitor progress
- Identify deficiencies
- Ask the learner, half way through the attachment, to do a self assessment of how things are going. If both you and the learner can identify deficiencies within a safe learning environment, you can work together to tackle them well before the attachment ends
- If you have serious concerns, you have an obligation to make them known to the learner and to the medical school or training authority
- It is not appropriate to diagnose serious problems and hand the learner on to the next stage of training in the hope that the problems will somehow be correct themselves

junior colleagues interact with a learner, you can encourage them with positive feedback on their teaching.

Every patient interview and every physical examination places the learner in a privileged relationship with a patient. We all have patients whom we especially admire—particularly people who have coped bravely with a chronic illness or a major disability, a disaster such as war, or other misfortunes. Such patients activate an emotional response in the learner, imprinting an enriched memory of the patient and the patient's illness.

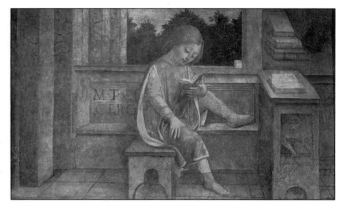

"Cultivate the society of the young, remain interested and never stop learning" (Cicero)

Promote active learning

- Time is limited in most clinical settings, and it can be tempting to revert to a passive observational teaching model
- Think about strategies to promote active learning
- Brief students to observe specific features of a consultation or procedure
- Ask patients for permission for the learner to carry out all or part of the physical examination or a procedure while you observe
- If space is available, allow students to interview patients in a separate room or cubicle before presenting them to you
- If possible videotape consultations for a debriefing session at a more convenient time
- Arrange for the learner to see the same patient over time, or in another context, such as a home visit

Reap the rewards

The role of the teacher is frequently undervalued, and yet teaching is potentially rewarding and enjoyable. It is also one of the defining features of a profession. Without teaching to ensure the transmission of knowledge, medicine becomes just another "job."

One to one teaching inevitably exposes you to evaluation by the learner. If the learner trusts you, he or she will be able to tell you what has worked well, and what could be improved. Respond to feedback by reflecting rather than by explaining, excusing, or offering counter arguments to defend your particular style. Openness to feedback is another professional attribute that is best modelled one to one.

Learners for whom you have been a role model and mentor are likely to repay you many times over. Sometimes you have the opportunity to observe their personal and professional development long after the one to one attachment has finished. Dr Sylvius knew how to do it, and Cicero understood its rejuvenating qualities.

Points to remember

Do
- Welcome
- Set shared achievable goals
- Put yourself in the learner's shoes
- Ask interesting questions
- Monitor progress and give feedback
- Encourage

Don't
- Appear unprepared
- Be vague about your expectations
- Confine the learner to passive roles
- Be "nit-picking"
- Leave feedback to the final assessment
- Humiliate

Further reading

- Parsell G, Bligh J. Recent perspectives on clinical teaching. *Med Educ* 2001;35:409-14.
- Paulman PM, Susman JL, Abboud CA, eds. *Precepting medical students in the office*. London: Johns Hopkins University Press, 2000.
- Westberg J, Jason H. *Collaborative clinical education: the foundation of effective health care*. New York: Springer, 1993.
- Whitehouse C, Roland M, Campion P, eds. *Teaching medicine in the community: a guide for undergraduate education*. New York: Oxford University Press, 1997.
- Stott N, Davis R. The exceptional potential in each primary care consultation. *J R Coll Gen Pract* 1979;29:201-5.
- Ausubel D, Novak J, Hanesian H. *Educational psychology: a cognitive view*. New York: Rinehart and Winston, 1978.

The illustration on p 544 is reproduced with permission from Jake Wyman/Photonica.

The illustration of the young Cicero reading (by Vicenzo Foppa) is reproduced with permission from the Bridgeman Art Library.

8 Learning and teaching in the clinical environment

John Spencer

Clinical teaching—that is, teaching and learning focused on, and usually directly involving, patients and their problems—lies at the heart of medical education. At undergraduate level, medical schools strive to give students as much clinical exposure as possible; they are also increasingly giving students contact with patients earlier in the course. For postgraduates, "on the job" clinical teaching is the core of their professional development. How can a clinical teacher optimise the teaching and learning opportunities that arise in daily practice?

Strengths, problems, and challenges

Learning in the clinical environment has many strengths. It is focused on real problems in the context of professional practice. Learners are motivated by its relevance and through active participation. Professional thinking, behaviour, and attitudes are "modelled" by teachers. It is the only setting in which the skills of history taking, physical examination, clinical reasoning, decision making, empathy, and professionalism can be taught and learnt as an integrated whole. Despite these potential strengths, clinical teaching has been much criticised for its variability, lack of intellectual challenge, and haphazard nature. In other words, clinical teaching is an educationally sound approach, all too frequently undermined by problems of implementation.

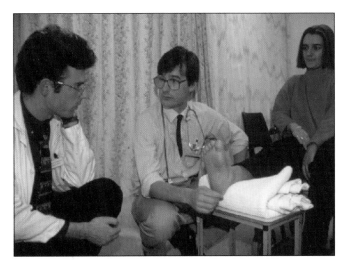
Clinical teaching in general practice

Common problems with clinical teaching

- Lack of clear objectives and expectations
- Focus on factual recall rather than on development of problem solving skills and attitudes
- Teaching pitched at the wrong level (usually too high)
- Passive observation rather than active participation of learners
- Inadequate supervision and provision of feedback
- Little opportunity for reflection and discussion
- "Teaching by humiliation"
- Informed consent not sought from patients
- Lack of respect for privacy and dignity of patients
- Lack of congruence or continuity with the rest of the curriculum

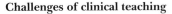

Challenges of clinical teaching

- Time pressures
- Competing demands—clinical (especially when needs of patients and students conflict); administrative; research
- Often opportunistic—makes planning more difficult
- Increasing numbers of students
- Fewer patients (shorter hospital stays; patients too ill or frail; more patients refusing consent)
- Often under-resourced
- Clinical environment not "teaching friendly" (for example, hospital ward)
- Rewards and recognition for teachers poor

The importance of planning

Many principles of good teaching, however, can (and should) be incorporated into clinical teaching. One of the most important is the need for planning. Far from compromising spontaneity, planning provides structure and context for both teacher and students, as well as a framework for reflection and evaluation. Preparation is recognised by students as evidence of a good clinical teacher.

How doctors teach

Almost all doctors are involved in clinical teaching at some point in their careers, and most undertake the job conscientiously and enthusiastically.

However, few receive any formal training in teaching skills, and in the past there has been an assumption that if a person simply knows a lot about their subject, they will be able to teach it. In reality, of course, although subject expertise is important, it

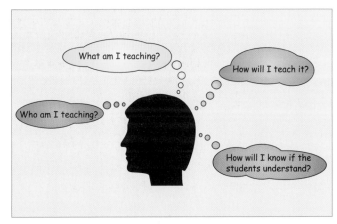
Questions to ask yourself when planning a clinical teaching session

is not sufficient. Effective clinical teachers use several distinct, if overlapping, forms of knowledge.

How students learn

Understanding the learning process will help clinical teachers to be more effective. Several theories are relevant (see first article in the series, 25 January). All start with the premise that learning is an active process (and, by inference, that the teacher's role is to act as facilitator). Cognitive theories argue that learning involves processing information through interplay between existing knowledge and new knowledge. An important influencing factor is what the learner knows already. The quality of the resulting new knowledge depends not only on "activating" this prior knowledge but also on the degree of elaboration that takes place. The more elaborate the resulting knowledge, the more easily it will be retrieved, particularly when learning takes place in the context in which the knowledge will be used.

Experiential learning

Experiential learning theory holds that learning is often most effective when based on experience. Several models have been described, the common feature being a cyclical process linking concrete experience with abstract conceptualisation through reflection and planning. Reflection is standing back and thinking about experience (What did it mean? How does it relate to previous experience? How did I feel?). Planning involves anticipating the application of new theories and skills (What will I do next time?). The experiential learning cycle, which can be entered at any stage, provides a useful framework for planning teaching sessions.

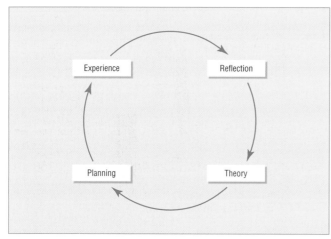

Experiential learning cycle: the role of the teacher is to help students to move round, and complete, the cycle

Questions

Questions may fulfil many purposes, such as to clarify understanding, to promote curiosity, and to emphasise key points. They can be classified as "closed," "open," and "clarifying" (or "probing") questions.

Closed questions invoke relatively low order thinking, often simple recall. Indeed, a closed question may elicit no response at all (for example, because the learner is worried about being wrong), and the teacher may end up answering their own question.

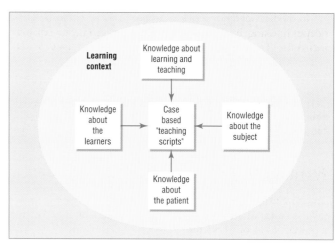

Various domains of knowledge contribute to the idiosyncratic teaching strategies ("teaching scripts") that tutors use in clinical settings

---

How to use cognitive learning theory in clinical teaching

Help students to identify what they already know
- "Activate" prior knowledge through brainstorming and briefing

Help students elaborate their knowledge
- Provide a bridge between existing and new information—for example, use of clinical examples, comparisons, analogies
- Debrief the students afterwards
- Promote discussion and reflection
- Provide relevant but variable contexts for the learning

Example of clinical teaching session based on experiential learning cycle

Setting—Six third year medical students doing introductory clinical skills course based in general practice

Topic—History taking and physical examination of patients with musculoskeletal problems (with specific focus on rheumatoid arthritis); three patients with good stories and signs recruited from the community

The session

Planning—Brainstorm for relevant symptoms and signs: this activates prior knowledge and orientates and provides framework and structure for the task

Experience—Students interview patients in pairs and do focused physical examination under supervision: this provides opportunities to implement and practise skills

Reflection—Case presentations and discussion: feedback and discussion provides opportunities for elaboration of knowledge

Theory—Didactic input from teacher (basic clinical information about rheumatoid arthritis): this links practice with theory

Planning— "What have I learned?" and "How will I approach such a patient next time?" Such questions prepare students for the next encounter and enable evaluation of the session

---

Effective teaching depends crucially on the teacher's communication skills. Two important areas of communication for effective teaching are questioning and giving explanations. Both are underpinned by attentive listening (including sensitivity to learners' verbal and non-verbal cues). It is important to allow learners to articulate areas in which they are having difficulties or which they wish to know more about

In theory, open questions are more likely to promote deeper thinking, but if they are too broad they may be equally ineffective. The purpose of clarifying and probing questions is self evident.

> Questions can be sequenced to draw out contributions or be built on to promote thinking at higher cognitive levels and to develop new understanding

Explanation

Teaching usually involves a lot of explanation, ranging from the (all too common) short lecture to "thinking aloud." The latter is a powerful way of "modelling" professional thinking, giving the novice insight into experts' clinical reasoning and decision making (not easily articulated in a didactic way). There are close analogies between teacher-student and doctor-patient communication, and the principles for giving clear explanations apply. If in doubt, pitch things at a low level and work upwards. As the late Sydney Jacobson, a journalist, said, "Never underestimate the person's intelligence, but don't overestimate their knowledge." Not only does a good teacher avoid answering questions, but he or she also questions answers.

Exploiting teaching opportunities

Most clinical teaching takes place in the context of busy practice, with time at a premium. Many studies have shown that a disproportionate amount of time in teaching sessions may be spent on regurgitation of facts, with relatively little on checking, probing, and developing understanding. Models for using time more effectively and efficiently and integrating teaching into day to day routines have been described. One such, the "one-minute preceptor," comprises a series of steps, each of which involves an easily performed task, which when combined form an integrated teaching strategy.

Teaching on the wards

Despite a long and worthy tradition, the hospital ward is not an ideal teaching venue. None the less, with preparation and forethought, learning opportunities can be maximised with minimal disruption to staff, patients, and their relatives.

Approaches include teaching on ward rounds (either dedicated teaching rounds or during "business" rounds); students seeing patients on their own (or in pairs—students can learn a lot from each other) then reporting back, with or without a follow up visit to the bedside for further discussion; and shadowing, when learning will inevitably be more opportunistic.

Key issues are careful selection of patients; ensuring ward staff know what's happening; briefing patients as well as students; using a side room (rather than the bedside) for discussions about patients; and ensuring that all relevant information (such as records and *x* ray films) is available.

Teaching in the clinic

Although teaching during consultations is organisationally appealing and minimally disruptive, it is limited in what it can achieve if students remain passive observers.

With relatively little impact on the running of a clinic, students can participate more actively. For example, they can be

How to use questions

- Restrict use of closed questions to establishing facts or baseline knowledge (What? When? How many?)
- Use open or clarifying/probing questions in all other circumstances (What are the options? What if?)
- Allow adequate time for students to give a response—don't speak too soon
- Follow a poor answer with another question
- Resist the temptation to answer learners' questions—use counter questions instead
- Statements make good questions—for example, "students sometimes find this difficult to understand" instead of "Do you understand?" (which may be intimidating)
- Be non-confrontational—you don't need to be threatening to be challenging

How to give effective explanations

- Check understanding before you start, as you proceed, and at the end—non-verbal cues may tell you all you need to know about someone's grasp of the topic
- Give information in "bite size" chunks
- Put things in a broader context when appropriate
- Summarise periodically ("so far, we've covered …") and at the end; asking learners to summarise is a powerful way of checking their understanding
- Reiterate the take home messages; again, asking students will give you feedback on what has been learnt (but be prepared for some surprises)

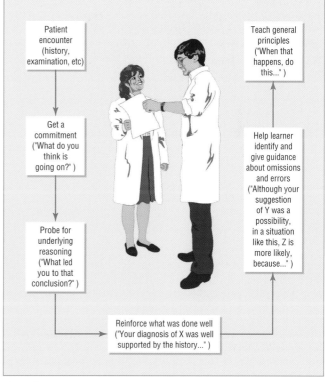

"One-minute preceptor" model

> Teaching during consultations has been much criticised for not actively involving learners

asked to make specific observations, write down thoughts about differential diagnosis or further tests, or note any questions—for discussion between patients. A more active approach is "hot seating." Here, the student leads the consultation, or part of it. His or her findings can be checked with the patient, and discussion and feedback can take place during or after the encounter. Students, although daunted, find this rewarding. A third model is when a student sees a patient alone in a separate room, and is then joined by the tutor. The student then presents their findings, and discussion follows. A limitation is that the teacher does not see the student in action. It also inevitably slows the clinic down, although not as much as might be expected. In an ideal world it would always be sensible to block out time in a clinic to accommodate teaching.

The patient's role

Sir William Osler's dictum that "it is a safe rule to have no teaching without a patient for a text, and the best teaching is that taught by the patient himself" is well known. The importance of learning from the patient has been repeatedly emphasised. For example, generations of students have been exhorted to "listen to the patient—he is telling you the diagnosis." Traditionally, however, a patient's role has been essentially passive, the patient acting as interesting teaching material, often no more than a medium through which the teacher teaches. As well as being potentially disrespectful, this is a wasted opportunity. Not only can patients tell their stories and show physical signs, but they can also give deeper and broader insights into their problems. Finally, they can give feedback to both learners and teacher. Through their interactions with patients, clinical teachers—knowingly or unknowingly—have a powerful influence on learners as role models.

Drs Gabrielle Greveson and Gail Young gave helpful feedback on early drafts.

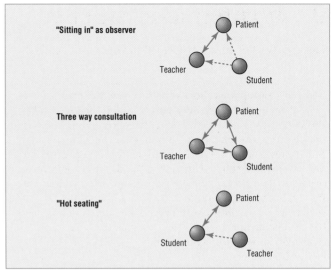

Seating arrangements for teaching in clinic or surgery

Working effectively and ethically with patients

- Think carefully about which parts of the teaching session require direct patient contact—is it necessary to have a discussion at the bedside?
- Always obtain consent from patients before the students arrive
- Ensure that students respect the confidentiality of all information relating to the patient, verbal or written
- Brief the patient before the session—purpose of the teaching session, level of students' experience, how the patient is expected to participate
- If appropriate, involve the patient in the teaching as much as possible
- Ask the patient for feedback—about communication and clinical skills, attitudes, and bedside manner
- Debrief the patient after the session—they may have questions, or sensitive issues may have been raised

Suggested reading

- Cox K. Planning bedside teaching. (Parts 1 to 8.) *Med J Australia* 1993;158:280-2, 355-7, 417-8, 493-5, 571-2, 607-8, 789-90, and 159:64-5.
- Parsell G, Bligh J. Recent perspectives on clinical teaching. *Med Educ* 2001;35:409-14.
- Hargreaves DH, Southworth GW, Stanley P, Ward SJ. *On-the-job learning for physicians.* London: Royal Society of Medicine, 1997.

9 Written assessment

Lambert W T Schuwirth, Cees P M van der Vleuten

Some misconceptions about written assessment may still exist, despite being disproved repeatedly by many scientific studies. Probably the most important misconception is the belief that the format of the question determines what the question actually tests. Multiple choice questions, for example, are often believed to be unsuitable for testing the ability to solve medical problems. The reasoning behind this assumption is that all a student has to do in a multiple choice question is recognise the correct answer, whereas in an open ended question he or she has to generate the answer spontaneously. Research has repeatedly shown, however, that the question's format is of limited importance and that it is the content of the question that determines almost totally what the question tests.

This does not imply that question formats are always interchangeable—some knowledge cannot be tested with multiple choice questions, and some knowledge is best not tested with open ended questions.

Five criteria can be used to evaluate the advantages and disadvantages of question types: reliability, validity, educational impact, cost effectiveness, and acceptability. Reliability pertains to the accuracy with which a score on a test is determined. Validity refers to whether the question actually tests what it is purported to test.

Educational impact is important because students tend to focus strongly on what they believe will be in the examinations. Therefore they will prepare strategically depending on the question types used. Whether different preparation leads to different types of knowledge is not fully clear, however. When teachers are forced to use a particular question type, they will tend to ask about the themes that can be easily assessed with that question type, and they will neglect the topics for which the question type is less well suited. Therefore, it is wise to vary the question types in different examinations.

Cost effectiveness and acceptability are important as the costs of different examinations have to be taken into account, and even the best designed examination will not survive if it is not accepted by teachers and students.

"True or false" questions

The main advantage of "true or false" questions is their conciseness. A question can be answered quickly by the student, so the test can cover a broad domain. Such questions, however, have two major disadvantages. Firstly, they are quite difficult to construct flawlessly—the statements have to be defensibly true or absolutely false. Teachers must be taught thoroughly how to construct these question types. Secondly, when a student answers a "false" question correctly, we can conclude only that the student knew the statement was false, not that he or she knew the correct fact.

"Single, best option" multiple choice questions

Multiple choice questions are well known, and there is extensive experience worldwide in constructing them. Their main advantage is the high reliability per hour of testing—mainly

> Choosing the most appropriate type of written examination for a certain purpose is often difficult. This article discusses some general issues of written assessment then gives an overview of the most commonly used types, together with their major advantages and disadvantages

Reliability

- A score that a student obtains on a test should indicate the score that this student would obtain in any other given (equally difficult) test in the same field ("parallel test")
- A test represents at best a sample—selected from a range of possible questions. So if a student passes a particular test one has to be sure that he or she would not have failed a parallel test, and vice versa
- Two factors influence reliability negatively:

  Sample error—The number of items may be too small to provide a reproducible result

  Sample too narrow—If the questions focus only on a certain element, the scores cannot generalise to the whole discipline

Validity

- The validity of a test is the extent to which it measures what it purports to measure
- Most competencies cannot be observed directly (body length, for example, can be observed directly; intelligence has to be derived from observations). Therefore, in examinations it is important to collect evidence to ensure validity:

  One simple piece of evidence could be, for example, that experts score higher than students on the test

  Alternative approaches include (a) an analysis of the distribution of course topics within test elements (a so called blueprint) and (b) an assessment of the soundness of individual test items.

- Good validation of tests should use several different pieces of evidence

> True or false questions are most suitable when the purpose of the question is to test whether students are able to evaluate the correctness of an assumption; in other cases they are best avoided

> Multiple choice questions can be used in any form of testing, except when spontaneous generation of the answer is essential, such as in creativity, hypothesising, and writing skills

because they are quick to answer—so a broad domain can be covered. They are often easier to construct than true or false questions and are more versatile. If constructed well, multiple choice questions can test more than simple facts. Unfortunately though, they are often used to test only facts, as teachers often think this is all they are fit for.

Multiple true or false questions

These questions enable the teacher to ask a question to which there is more than one correct answer. Although they take somewhat longer to answer than the previous two types, their reliability per hour of testing time is not much lower.

Construction, however, is not easy. It is important to have sufficient distracters (incorrect options) and to find a good balance between the number of correct options and distracters. In addition, it is essential to construct the question so that correct options are defensibly correct and distracters are defensibly incorrect. A further disadvantage is the rather complicated scoring procedure for these questions.

"Short answer" open ended questions

Open ended questions are more flexible—in that they can test issues that require, for example, creativity, spontaneity—but they have lower reliability. Because answering open ended questions is much more time consuming than answering multiple choice questions, they are less suitable for broad sampling. They are also expensive to produce and to score. When writing open ended questions it is important to describe clearly how detailed the answer should be—without giving away the answer. A good open ended question should include a detailed answer key for the person marking the paper. Short answer, open ended questions are not suitable for assessing factual knowledge; use multiple choice questions instead.

Short answer, open ended questions should be aimed at the aspects of competence that cannot be tested in any other way.

Essays

Essays are ideal for assessing how well students can summarise, hypothesise, find relations, and apply known procedures to new situations. They can also provide an insight into different aspects of writing ability and the ability to process information. Unfortunately, answering them is time consuming, so their reliability is limited.

When constructing essay questions, it is essential to define the criteria on which the answers will be judged. A common pitfall is to "over-structure" these criteria in the pursuit of objectivity, and this often leads to trivialising the questions. Some structure and criteria are necessary, but too detailed a structure provides little gain in reliability and a considerable loss of validity. Essays involve high costs, so they should be used sparsely and only in cases where short answer, open ended questions or multiple choice questions are not appropriate.

"Key feature" questions

In such a question, a description of a realistic case is followed by a small number of questions that require only essential decisions; these questions may be either multiple choice or open ended, depending on the content of the question. Key feature questions seem to measure problem solving ability

> **Teachers need to be taught well how to write good multiple choice questions**

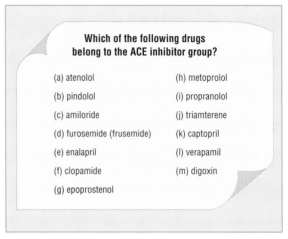

Which of the following drugs belong to the ACE inhibitor group?

(a) atenolol	(h) metoprolol
(b) pindolol	(i) propranolol
(c) amiloride	(j) triamterene
(d) furosemide (frusemide)	(k) captopril
(e) enalapril	(l) verapamil
(f) clopamide	(m) digoxin
(g) epoprostenol	

Example of a multiple, true or false question

> **Open ended questions are perhaps the most widely accepted question type. Their format is commonly believed to be intrinsically superior to a multiple choice format. Much evidence shows, however, that this assumed superiority is limited**

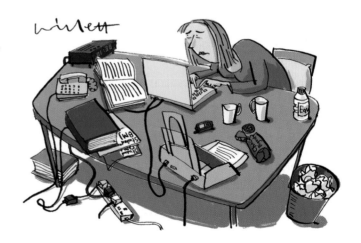

> **"Key feature" questions aim to measure problem solving ability validly without losing too much reliability**

validly and have good reliability. In addition, most people involved consider them to be a suitable approach, which makes them more acceptable.

However, the key feature approach is rather new and therefore less well known than the other approaches. Also, construction of the questions is time consuming; inexperienced teachers may need up to three hours to produce a single key feature case with questions. Experienced writers, though, may produce up to four an hour. Nevertheless, these questions are expensive to produce, and large numbers of cases are normally needed to prevent students from memorising cases. Key feature questions are best used for testing the application of knowledge and problem solving in "high stakes" examinations.

Extended matching questions

The key elements of extended matching questions are a list of options, a "lead-in" question, and some case descriptions or vignettes. Students should understand that an option may be correct for more than one vignette, and some options may not apply to any of the vignettes. The idea is to minimise the recognition effect that occurs in standard multiple choice questions because of the many possible combinations between vignettes and options. Also, by using cases instead of facts, the items can be used to test application of knowledge or problem solving ability. They are easier to construct than key feature questions, as many cases can be derived from one set of options. Their reliability has been shown to be good. Scoring of the answers is easy and could be done with a computer.

The format of extended matching questions is still relatively unknown, so teachers need training and practice before they can write these questions. There is a risk of an under-representation of certain themes simply because they do not fit the format. Extended matching questions are best used when large numbers of similar sorts of decisions (for example, relating to diagnosis or ordering of laboratory tests) need testing for different situations.

Conclusion

Choosing the best question type for a particular examination is not simple. A careful balancing of costs and benefits is required. A well designed assessment programme will use different types of question appropriate for the content being tested.

Further reading

- Case SM, Swanson DB. Extended-matching items: a practical alternative to free response questions. *Teach Learn Med* 1993;5:107-15.
- Frederiksen N. The real test bias: influences of testing on teaching and learning. *Am Psychol* 1984;39:193-202.
- Bordage G. An alternative approach to PMPs: the "key-features" concept. In: Hart IR, Harden R, eds. *Further developments in assessing clinical competence; proceedings of the second Ottawa conference.* Montreal: Can-Heal Publications, 1987:59-75.
- Swanson DB, Norcini JJ, Grosso LJ. Assessment of clinical competence: written and computer-based simulations. *Assessment and Evaluation in Higher Education* 1987;12:220-46.
- Ward WC. A comparison of free-response and multiple-choice forms of verbal aptitude tests. *Applied Psychological Measurement* 1982;6(1):1-11.
- Schuwirth LWT. *An approach to the assessment of medical problem solving: computerised case-based testing.* Maastricht: Datawyse Publications, 1998. (Thesis from Department of Educational Development and Research, Maastricht University.)

Example of a key feature question

Case

You are a general practitioner. Yesterday you made a house call on Mr Downing. From your history taking and physical examination you diagnosed nephrolithiasis. You gave an intramuscular injection of 100 mg diclofenac, and you left him some diclofenac suppositories. You advised him to take one when in pain but not more than two a day. Today he rings you at 9 am. He still has pain attacks, which respond well to the diclofenac, but since 5 am he has also had a continuous pain in his right side and a fever (38.9°C).

Which of the following is the best next step?
(a) Ask him to wait another day to see how the disease progresses
(b) Prescribe broad spectrum antibiotics
(c) Refer him to hospital for an intravenous pyelogram
(d) Refer him urgently to a urologist

Example of an extended matching question

(a) *Campylobacter jejuni*, (b) *Candida albicans*, (c) *Giardia lamblia*, (d) *Rotavirus*, (e) *Salmonella typhi*, (f) *Yersinia enterocolitica*, (g) *Pseudomonas aeruginosa*, (h) *Escherichia coli*, (i) *Helicobacter pylori*, (j) *Clostridium perfringens*, (k) *Mycobacterium tuberculosis*, (l) *Shigella flexneri*, (m) *Vibrio cholerae*, (n) *Clostridium difficile*, (o) *Proteus mirabilis*, (p) *Tropheryma whippelii*

For each of the following cases, select (from the list above) the micro-organism most likely to be responsible:
- A 48 year old man with a chronic complaint of dyspepsia suddenly develops severe abdominal pain. On physical examination there is general tenderness to palpation with rigidity and rebound tenderness. Abdominal radiography shows free air under the diaphragm
- A 45 year old woman is treated with antibiotics for recurring respiratory tract infections. She develops a severe abdominal pain with haemorrhagic diarrhoea. Endoscopically a pseudomembranous colitis is seen

---

Using only one type of question throughout the whole curriculum is not a valid approach

10 Skill based assessment

Sydney Smee

Skill based assessments are designed to measure the knowledge, skills, and judgment required for competency in a given domain. Assessment of clinical skills has formed a key part of medical education for hundreds of years. However, the basic requirements for reliability and validity have not always been achieved in traditional "long case" and "short case" assessments. Skill based assessments have to contend with case specificity, which is the variance in performance that occurs over different cases or problems. In other words, case specificity means that performance with one patient related problem does not reliably predict performance with subsequent problems.

For a reliable measure of clinical skills, performance has to be sampled across a range of patient problems. This is the basic principle underlying the development of objective structured clinical examinations (OSCEs). Several other structured clinical examinations have been developed in recent years, including modified OSCEs—such as the Royal College of Physicians' Practical Assessment of Clinical Examination Skills (PACES) and the objective structured long case (OSLER). This article focuses mainly on OSCEs to illustrate the principles of skill based assessment.

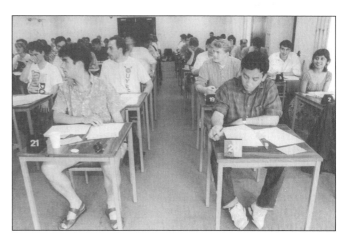

Written tests can assess knowledge acquisition and reasoning ability, but they cannot so easily measure skills

OSCEs

The objective structured clinical examination (OSCE) was introduced over 30 years ago as a reliable approach to assessing basic clinical skills. It is a flexible test format based on a circuit of patient based "stations."

At each station, trainees interact with a patient or a "standardised patient" to demonstrate specified skills. Standardised patients are lay people trained to present patient problems realistically. The validity of interactions with real patients, however, may be higher than that with standardised patients, but standardised patients are particularly valuable when communication skills are being tested.

OSCE stations may be short (for eample, five minutes) or long (15-30 minutes). There may be as few as eight stations or more than 20. Scoring is done with a task specific checklist or a combination of checklist and rating scale. The scoring of the students or trainees may be done by observers (for example, faculty members) or patients and standardised patients.

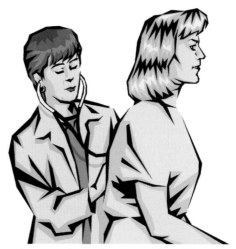

Patient-doctor interaction for assessing clinical performance

Design

The design of an OSCE is usually the result of a compromise between the assessment objectives and logistical constraints; however, the content should always be linked to the curriculum, as this link is essential for validity.

Using many short stations should generate scores that are sufficiently reliable for making pass-fail decisions within a reasonable testing time. (Whether any OSCE is sufficiently reliable for grading decisions is debatable.) Fewer but longer stations maximise learning relative to the selected patient problems, especially when students or trainees receive feedback on their performance. The number of students, time factors, and the availability of appropriate space must also be considered.

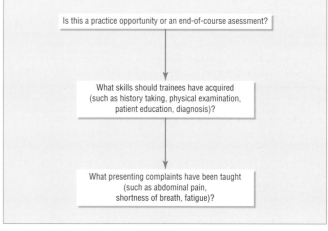

Is this a practice opportunity or an end-of-course asessment?

↓

What skills should trainees have acquired (such as history taking, physical examination, patient education, diagnosis)?

↓

What presenting complaints have been taught (such as abdominal pain, shortness of breath, fatigue)?

Questions to answer when designing an OSCE

Planning

Planning is critical. Patients and standardised patients can be recruited only after stations are written. Checklists must be reviewed before being printed, and their format must be compatible with the marking method, ideally computerised. OSCEs generate a lot of data—for 120 students in a 20 station OSCE there will be 2400 mark sheets!)

Stations are the backbone of an OSCE, and yet the single most common problem is that station materials are incomplete and subject to last minute changes. The result is increased cost and wasted time.

If OSCE scores are being used for making pass-fail decisions, then it is also necessary to set strandards. Several methods for setting standards have been used, with the Angoff method described below being the most commonly used.

Plans should allow sufficient time to process and analyse the scores carefully.

Costs

OSCE costs vary greatly because the number of stations determines the number of standardised patients, examiners, and staff required. Whether or not faculty members volunteer to write cases, set standards, and examine is also a significant factor.

Developing the stations

OSCE stations have three components.

Stem

A standardised format for the "stem" (task) is helpful—for example, providing the patient's name, age, presenting complaint, and the setting (such as clinic, emergency, or ward) for all stations. The stem must clearly state the task—for example, "in the next eight minutes, conduct a relevant physical examination."

Checklist

The checklist items are the actions that should be taken in response to the information in the stem. These items should be reviewed and edited to ensure that (a) they are appropriate for the level of training being assessed, (b) they are task based, and (c) they are observable (so the observer can score them).

The length of the checklist depends on the clinical task, the time allowed, and who is scoring. A checklist for a five minute station that is testing history taking may have up to 25 items if a faculty observer is doing the scoring. If a patient or standardised patient is doing the scoring, then fewer items should be used. Use of detailed items will guide scorers: for example, "examines the abdomen" is a general item that might better be separated into a series of items such as "inspects the abdomen," "auscultates the abdomen," "lightly palpates all four quadrants," and so on.

A score must be assigned to every item. Items may be scored 1 or 0, or relative weights may be assigned, with more critical items being worth more. Weights may not change the overall pass-fail rate of an OSCE, but they may improve the validity of a checklist and can affect which trainees pass or fail.

Training information

For standardised patients, directions should use patient based language, specify the patient's perception of the problem (for example, serious, not serious), provide only relevant information, and specify pertinent negatives. Responses to all checklist items should be included. The patient's behaviour and affect should be described in terms of body language, verbal

Tasks to do ahead

- Create blueprint
- Set timeline (how long do we need?)
- Get authors for a case-writing workshop
- Review and finalise cases
- Arrange workshop on setting standards
- Recruit standardised patients; recruit faculty members as examiners
- Train standardised patients
- Print marking sheets, make signs
- List all supplies for set-up of OSCE stations
- Remind everyone of date
- Make sure students have all the information
- Plans for the examination day: diagram of station layout; directions for examiners, standardised patients, and staff; possible registration table for students; timing and signals (for example, stopwatch and whistles); procedures for ending the examination
- Anything else?

> The fixed costs of running an OSCE remain much the same regardless of the number of examination candidates. Administering an OSCE twice in one day only slightly increases the fixed costs, although the examiners' time is an important cost

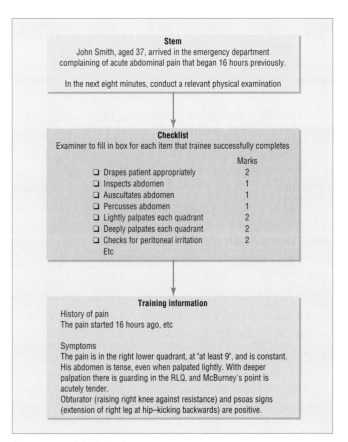

Components of OSCE station

tone, and pace. Symptoms to be simulated need to be described.

Limitations

Skill based assessments are based on tasks that approximate performance in the area of interest. The assumption is that the closer the tasks are to "real world" tasks, the more valid the assessment.

Three aspects of an OSCE limit how closely the stations approximate clinical practice. Firstly, time limited stations often require trainees to perform isolated aspects of the clinical encounter. This deconstructs the doctor-patient encounter and may be unacceptable for formative assessments. The trade-off is that limiting the time allows for more stations, which can provide performance snapshots that allow for reliable, summative decision making.

Secondly, OSCEs rely on task specific checklists, which assume that the doctor-patient interaction can be described as a list of actions. As a result, checklists tend to emphasise thoroughness, and this may become a less relevant criterion as the clinical experience of candidates increases. Thirdly, there are limits to what can be simulated, and this constrains the nature of the patient problems that can be sampled. Again, this becomes more of an issue as candidates' level of training and clinical experience increases.

Other approaches to skill based assessment

Traditional approaches

The oral examination (also known as the "viva") and the "long case" have long been used for assessing clinical competence. The oral examination is traditionally an unstructured face to face session with the examiners. This allows them to explore the trainee's understanding of topics deemed relevant to clinical practice. The long case is patient based, but the interaction with the patient is usually not observed. Instead, trainees summarise the patient problem for the examiners and respond to examiners' questions about findings, diagnosis or management, and other topics deemed relevant by examiners. The strength of the long case is the validity that comes from the complexities of a complete encounter with a real patient. However, the difficulty and relevance of these assessments varies greatly as the content is limited to one or two patient problems (selected from the available patients), and decisions are made according to unknown criteria, as examiners make holistic judgments. For this reason traditional unstructured orals and long cases have largely been discontinued in North America.

Alternative formats

Alternative formats tackle the problems associated with traditional orals and long cases by (a) having examiners observe the candidate's complete interaction with the patient, (b) training examiners to a structured assessment process, and/or (c) increasing the number of patient problems. For a short case assessment, for example, one or two examiners may direct a trainee through a series of five or six encounters with real patients. They observe, ask questions, and make a judgment based on the candidate's performance with all the patients. Similarly, a structured oral examination is still a face to face session with examiners, but guidelines for the topics to be covered are provided. Alternatively, a series of patient scenarios and agreed questions may be used so that the content and difficulty of the assessment is standardised across the trainees. Each of these adaptations is aimed at improving reliability, but

Limitations of OSCEs
- Stations often require trainees to perform isolated aspects of the clinical encounter, which "deconstructs" the doctor-patient encounter
- OSCEs rely on task specific checklists, which tend to emphasise thoroughness. But with increasing experience, thoroughness becomes less relevant
- The limitations on what can be simulated constrain the type of patient problems that can be used

None of these limitations is prohibitive, but they should be considered when selecting an OSCE as an assessment tool and when making inferences from OSCE scores

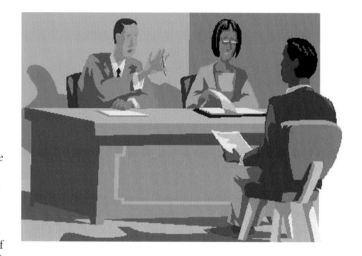

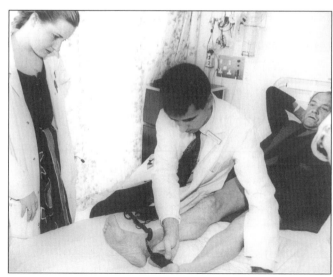

An alternative way to assess skills is to observe candidates' interaction with patients

the most important improvement comes from greatly increasing the number of patient problems, which may well cause an impractical increased testing time.

Reliability and validity

The reliability of a test describes the degree to which the test consistently measures what it is supposed to measure. The more reliable a test, the more likely it is that a similar result will be obtained if the test is readministered. Reliability is sensitive to the length of the test, the station or item discrimination, and the heterogeneity of the cohort of candidates. Standardised patients' portrayals, patients' behaviour, examiners' behaviour, and administrative variables also affect reliability.

The validity of a test is a measure of the degree to which the test actually measures what it is supposed to measure. Validity is a property of test scores and justifies their interpretation for a specific purpose. The most basic evidence of validity comes from documenting the links between the content of the assessment and the curriculum's objectives and from the qualifications of those who develop the assessment.

Setting standards

Checklists generate scores; judges set standards. The validity of a standard depends on the judges' qualifications and the reasonableness of the procedure they use to set it. When pass-fail decisions are being made, a skill based assessment should be "criterion referenced" (that is, trainees should be assessed relative to performance standards rather than to each other or to a reference group). An Angoff approach is commonly used to set the standard for an OSCE.

Skill based assessments do not replace knowledge based tests, but they do assess aspects of competence that knowledge based tests cannot assess. Although the use of OSCEs for skill based assessment is increasingly widespread, modifying more traditional formats may be appropriate when they are combined with other forms of assessment or are used to screen trainees. The success of any skill based assessment depends on finding a suitable balance between validity and reliability and between the ideal and the practical.

Factors leading to lower reliability

- Too few stations or too little testing time
- Checklists or items that don't discriminate (that is, are too easy or too hard)
- Unreliable patients or inconsistent portrayals by standardised patients
- Examiners who score idiosyncratically
- Administrative problems (such as disorganised staff or noisy rooms)

Questions to ensure validity

- Are the patient problems relevant and important to the curriculum?
- Will the stations assess skills that have been taught?
- Have content experts (generalists and specialists) reviewed the stations?

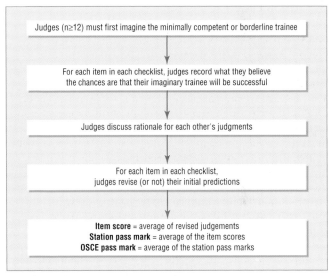

A modified Angoff procedure for an OSCE

The second picture and the picture showing an oral examination are from Microsoft Clipart.

Further reading

- Gorter S, Rethans JJ, Scherpbier A, van der Heijde D, Houben H, van der Linden S, et al. Developing case-specific checklists for standardized-patient-based assessments in internal medicine: a review of the literature. *Acad Med* 2000;75:1130-7.
- Hodges B, Regehr G, McNaughton N, Tiberius RG, Hanson M. OSCE checklists do not capture increasing levels of expertise. *Acad Med* 1999;74:1129-34.
- Kaufman DM, Mann KV, Muijtjens AMM, van der Vleuten CPM. A comparison of standard-setting procedures for an OSCE in undergraduate medical education. *Acad Med* 2001;75:267-71.
- Newble DI, Dawson B, Dauphinee WD, Page G, Macdonald M, Swanson DB, et al. Guidelines for assessing clinical competence. *Teach Learn Med* 1994;6:213-20.
- Norcini JJ. The death of the long case? *BMJ* 2002;324:408-9.
- Reznick RK, Smee SM, Baumber JS, Cohen R, Rothman AI, Blackmore DE, et al. Guidelines for estimating the real cost of an objective structured clinical examination. *Acad Med* 1993;67:513-7.

11 Work based assessment

John J Norcini

In 1990 psychologist George Miller proposed a framework for assessing clinical competence. At the lowest level of the pyramid is knowledge (knows), followed by competence (knows how), performance (shows how), and action (does). In this framework, Miller distinguished between "action" and the lower levels. "Action" focuses on what occurs in practice rather than what happens in an artificial testing situation. Work based methods of assessment target this highest level of the pyramid and collect information about doctors' performance in their normal practice. Other common methods of assessment, such as multiple choice questions, simulation tests, and objective structured clinical examinations (OSCEs) target the lower levels of the pyramid. Underlying this distinction is the sensible but still unproved assumption that assessments of actual practice are a much better reflection of routine performance than assessments done under test conditions.

Methods

Although the focus of this article is on practising doctors, work based assessment methods apply to medical students and trainees as well. These methods can be classified in many ways, but this article classifies them in two dimensions. The first dimension describes the basis for making judgments about the quality of performance. The second dimension is concerned with how data are collected.

Basis for judgment

Outcomes

In judgments about the outcomes of their patients, the quality of a cardiologist, for example, might be judged by the mortality of his or her patients within 30 days of acute myocardial infarction. Historically, outcomes have been limited to mortality and morbidity, but in recent years the number of clinical end points has been expanded. Patients' satisfaction, functional status, cost effectiveness, and intermediate outcomes—for example, HbA_{1c} and lipid concentrations for diabetic patients—have gained acceptance.

Patients' outcomes are the best measures of the quality of doctors for the public, the patients, and doctors themselves. For the public, outcomes assessment is a measure of accountability that provides reassurance that the doctor is performing well in practice. For individual patients, it supplies a basis for deciding which doctor to see. For doctors, it offers reassurance that their assessment is tailored to their unique practice and based on real work performance.

Despite the fact that an assessment of outcomes is highly desirable, at least four substantial problems remain. These are attribution, complexity, case mix, and numbers.

Firstly, for a good judgment to be made about a doctor's performance, the patients' outcomes must be attributable solely to that doctor's actions. This is not realistic when care is delivered within systems and teams. Secondly, patients with the same condition will vary in complexity depending on the severity of their illness, the existence of comorbid conditions, and their ability to comply with the doctor's recommendations. Although statistical adjustments may tackle these problems, they are not completely effective. So differences in complexity directly influence outcomes and make it difficult to compare

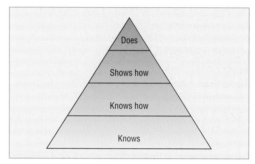

This article explains what is meant by work based assessment and presents a classification scheme for current methods

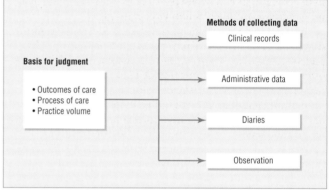

Miller's pyramid for assessing clinical competence

Classification for work based assessment methods

Three aspects of doctors' performance can be assessed—patients' outcomes, process of care, and volume of practice

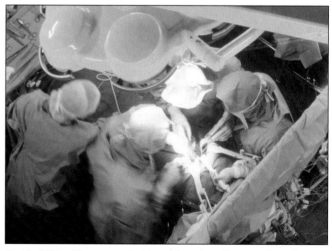

Care is delivered in teams, so judging a doctor's performance through outcomes is not realistic

doctors or set standards for their performance. Thirdly, unevenness exists in the case mix of different doctors, again making it difficult to compare performance or to set standards. Finally, to estimate well a doctor's routine performance, a sizeable number of patients are needed. This limits outcomes assessment to the most frequently occurring conditions.

Process of care

In judgments about the process of care that doctors provide, a general practitioner, for example, might be assessed on the basis of how many of his or her patients aged over 50 years have been screened for colorectal cancer. General process measures include screening, preventive services, diagnosis, management, prescribing, education of patients, and counselling. In addition, condition specific processes might also serve as the basis for making judgments about doctors—for example, whether diabetic patients have their HbA_{1c} monitored regularly and receive routine foot examinations.

Measures of process of care have substantial advantages over outcomes. Firstly, the process of care is more directly in the control of the doctor, so problems of attribution are greatly reduced. Secondly, the measures are less influenced by the complexity of patients' problems—for example, doctors continue to monitor HbA_{1c} regardless of the severity of the diabetes. Thirdly, some of the process measures, such as immunisation, should be offered to all patients of a particular type, reducing the problems of case mix.

The major disadvantage of process measures is that simply doing the right thing does not ensure the best outcomes for patients. That a physician regularly monitors HbA_{1c}, for example, does not guarantee that he or she will make the necessary changes in management. Furthermore, although process measures are less susceptible to the difficulties of attribution, complexity, and case mix, these factors still have an adverse influence.

Volume

Judgments about the number of times that doctors have engaged in a particular activity might include, for example, the number of times a surgeon performed a certain surgical procedure. The premise for this type of assessment is the large body of research showing that quality of care is associated with higher volume.

Data collection

Clinical practice records

One of the best sources of information about outcomes, process, and volume is the clinical practice record. The external audit of these records is a valid and credible source of data. Two major problems exist, however, with clinical practice records.

Firstly, judgment can be made only on what is recorded —this may not be an accurate assessment of what was actually done in practice.

Secondly, abstracting records is expensive and time consuming and is made cumbersome by the fact that they are often incomplete or illegible.

Widespread adoption of the electronic medical record may be the ultimate solution, although this is some years away. Meanwhile, some groups rely on doctors to abstract their own records and submit them for evaluation. Coupled with an external audit of a sample of the participating doctors, this is a credible and feasible alternative.

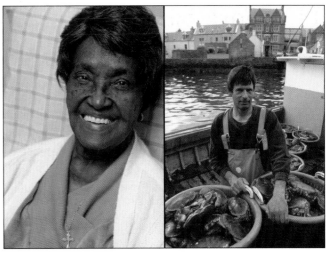

Unevenness in case mix can reduce usefulness of using patients' outcomes as a measure of doctors' competence

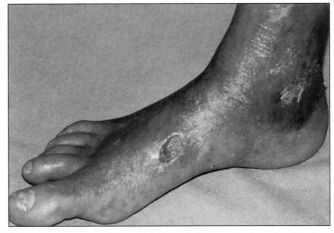

Judgments on process of care might include foot examinations for diabetic patients

> **For a sound assessment of an individual doctor's process of care, a sizeable number of patients need to be included**

Advantages of volume based assessment over assessment of outcomes and process

- Problems of attribution are reduced substantially
- Complexity is eliminated
- Case mix is not relevant

However, such assessment alone offers no assurance that the activity was conducted properly

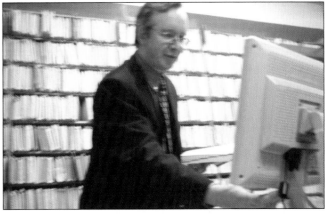

Traditional medical records may give way to widespread use of electronic records, making data collection easier and quicker

Administrative databases

In some healthcare systems large computerised databases are often developed as part of the process of administering and reimbursing for health care. Data from these sources are accessible, inexpensive, and widely available. They can be used in the evaluation of some aspects of practice performance—such as cost effectiveness—and of medical errors. However, the lack of clinical information and the fact that the data are often collected for invoicing purposes makes them unsuitable as the only source of information.

Diaries

Doctors, especially trainees, may use diaries or logs to record the procedures they perform. Depending on the purpose of the diary, entries can be accompanied by a description of the doctor's role, the name of an observer, an indication of whether it was done properly, and a list of complications. This is a reasonable way to collect data on volume and an acceptable alternative to the abstraction of clinical practice records until medical records are kept electronically.

Observation

Data can be collected in many ways through practice observation, but to be consistent with Miller's definition of work based assessment, the observations need to be routine or covert to avoid an artificial test situation. They can be made in any number of ways and by any number of different observers. The most common forms of observation based assessment are ratings by supervisors, peers, and patients. Other examples of observation include visits by standardised patients (lay people trained to present patient problems realistically) to doctors in their surgeries and audiotapes or videotapes of consultations such as those used by the General Medical Council.

Portfolios

Doctors typically collect from various sources the practice data they think pertinent to their evaluation. A doctor's portfolio might contain data on outcomes, process, or volume, collected through clinical record audit, diaries, or assessments by patients and peers. It is important to specify what to include in portfolios as doctors will naturally present their best work, and the evaluation of it will not be useful for continuing quality improvement or quality assurance. In addition, if there is a desire to compare doctors or to provide them with feedback about their relative performance, then all portfolios must contain the same data collected in a similar fashion. Otherwise, there is no basis for legitimate comparison or benchmarking.

Further reading

- McKinley RK, Fraser RC, Baker R. Model for directly assessing and improving competence and performance in revalidation of clinicians. *BMJ* 2001;322:712-5.
- Miller GE. The assessment of clinical skills/competence/performance. *Acad Med* 1990:S63-7.
- Norcini JJ. Recertification in the United States. *BMJ* 1999;319:1183-5.
- Cunningham JPW, Hanna E, Turnbull J, Kaigas T, Norman GR. Defensible assessment of the competency of the practicing physician. *Acad Med* 1997;72:9-12.

> **Databases for clinical audit are becoming more available and may provide more useful information relating to clinical practice**

Peer evaluation rating forms

Below are the aspects of competence assessed with the peer rating form developed by Ramsey and colleagues.* The form, given to 10 peers, provides reliable estimates of two overall dimensions of performance: cognitive and clinical skills, and professionalism.

Cognitive and clinical skills	Professionalism
• Medical knowledge	• Respect
• Ambulatory care	• Integrity
• Management of complex problems	• Psychosocial aspects of illness
• Management of hospital inpatients	• Compassion
• Problem solving	• Responsibility
• Overall clinical competence	

*Ramsey PG et al. Use of peer ratings to evaluate physician performance. *JAMA* 1993;269:1655-60

Patient rating form*

The form is given to 25 patients and gives a reliable estimate of a doctor's communication skills. Scores are on a five point scale—poor to excellent—and are related to validity measures. The patients must be balanced in terms of age, sex, and health status. Typical questions are:

- Tells you everything?
- Greets you warmly?
- Treats you as if you're on the same level?
- Lets you tell your story?
- Shows interest in you as a person?
- Warns you what is coming during the physical examination?
- Discusses options?
- Explains what you need to know?
- Uses words you can understand?

*Webster GD. *Final report of the patient satisfaction questionnaire study.* American Board of Internal Medicine, 1989

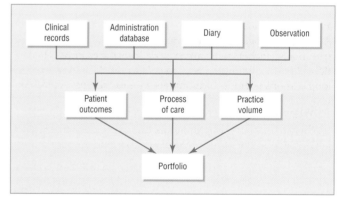

How portfolios are compiled

The photograph of a surgical team is from Philippe Plailly/Eurelios/SPL; the photographs illustrating case mix are from Photofusion, by David Tothill (left) and Pete Addis (right); the photograph of the foot is from Ray Clarke (FRPS) and Mervyn Goff (FRPS/SPL); and the medical records photograph is from Michael Donne/SPL.

12　Educational environment

Linda Hutchinson

A student might find a particular question threatening and intimidating in one context yet stimulating and challenging in a different context. What makes one learning context unpleasant and another pleasant?

Learning depends on several factors, but a crucial step is the engagement of the learner. This is affected by their motivation and perception of relevance. These, in turn, can be affected by learners' previous experiences and preferred learning styles and by the context and environment in which the learning is taking place. In adult learning theories, teaching is as much about setting the context or climate for learning as it is about imparting knowledge or sharing expertise.

Motivation

Motivation can be intrinsic (from the student) and extrinsic (from external factors). Assessments are usually a strong extrinsic motivator for learners. Individual learners' intrinsic motivation can be affected by previous experiences, by their desire to achieve, and the relevance of the learning to their future.

A teacher's role in motivation should not be underestimated. Enthusiasm for the subject, interest in the students' experiences, and clear direction (among other things) all help to keep students' attention and improve assimilation of information and understanding.

Even with good intrinsic motivation, however, external factors can demotivate and disillusion. Distractions, unhelpful attitudes of teachers, and physical discomfort will prompt learners to disengage. Maslow described a model to illustrate the building blocks of motivation. Each layer needs to be in place before the pinnacle of "self actualisation" is reached.

Physiological needs

Although the need to be fed, watered, and comfortable seems trite, many teachers will have experienced, for example, the difficulties of running sessions in cold or overheated rooms, in long sessions without refreshments, in noisy rooms, in facilities with uncomfortable seating.

Physical factors can make it difficult for learners and teachers to relax and pay attention. Ensuring adequate breaks and being mindful of the physical environment are part of the teacher's role.

Safety

A teacher should aim to provide an environment in which learners feel safe to experiment, voice their concerns, identify their lack of knowledge, and stretch their limits. Safety can be compromised, for example, through humiliation, harassment, and threat of forced disclosure of personal details.

Teachers can create an atmosphere of respect by endorsing the learners' level of knowledge and gaps in knowledge as essential triggers to learning rather than reasons for ridicule.

Remembering names and involving the learners in setting ground rules are other examples of building mutual trust. Feedback on performance, a vital part of teaching, should be done constructively and with respect for the learner.

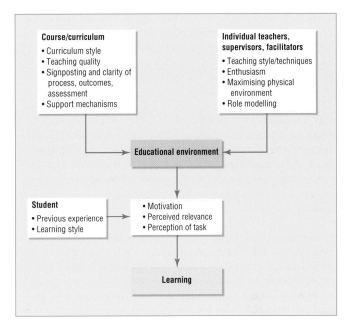

Many factors influence learning

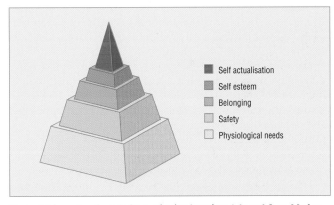

Maslow's hierarchy of needs for motivating learning. Adapted from Maslow A H. *Motivation and Personality*, New York: Harper and Row, 1954

Case history: safe environment

Dr Holden claims to use interactive teaching techniques. She introduces the topic then points to a student in the audience and says, "tell me five causes of cyanosis." Each student will get asked questions in the session, and most spend their time worrying about when it is their turn to be "exposed."

After a course on teaching skills, she runs the same session. After the introduction, she tells the students to turn to their neighbour and together come up with some possible causes of cyanosis. After a couple of minutes of this "buzz group" activity, she asks for one suggestion from each group until no new suggestions are made. The suggestions are then discussed with reference to the aims of the session.

Belonging

Many factors help to give a student a sense of belonging in a group or team—for example, being a respected member, having one's voice heard and attended to, being given a useful role, and having colleagues with similar backgrounds, experiences, and goals.

Learners are motivated through inclusion and consultation. Their input to a course's objectives and structure should be sought, valued, and acted on. On clinical placements, staff should help to prevent medical students from feeling ignored, marginalised, or "in the way." Students should instead be valued as assets to a clinical unit or team.

Self esteem

Several of the points mentioned above feed directly into self esteem through making the learner feel valued. Praise, words of appreciation, and constructive rather than destructive criticism are important. It can take many positive moments to build self esteem, but just one unkind and thoughtless comment to destroy it.

Doctors are well used to their role in the doctor-patient relationship. Some find it hard to translate the same skills and attitudes to the teacher-student relationship. Their own experience of education or their own distractions, time pressures, and other stresses may be factors.

Self actualisation

If a teacher has attended to the above motivational factors, then they have sought to provide the ideal environment in which a learner can flourish.

An ethos that encourages intrinsic motivation without anxiety is conducive to a "deep" learning approach. However, there may be some who remain unable to respond to the education on offer. Teachers may need to consider whether the course (or that particular piece of study) is suitable for that student.

Relevance

The relevance of learning is closely linked to motivation: relevance for immediate needs, for future work, of getting a certificate or degree regardless of content. Learning for learning's sake is back in vogue in higher education after a move towards vocational or industrial preparation.

Certain courses in medical degrees have been notoriously poorly received by students. Faculty members need to explain to students why these courses are necessary and how they link to future practice. Allowing them to see for themselves, through early clinical exposure and experience, is likely to be helpful. Similarly, learning the basic medical sciences in the context of clinical situations is the basis for problem based learning.

A challenging problem is the trainee who is in a post because he or she needs to do it for certification, although it is of no perceived value to the trainee's future career direction. A balance needs to be negotiated between respect for the individual's needs and the expectation of a level of professional conduct.

Teacher as role model

The teacher or facilitator is one of the most powerful variables in the educational environment. The teacher's actions, attitudes (as evidenced by tone of voice, comments made), enthusiasm, and interest in the subject will affect learners indirectly. The capacity for subliminal messages is enormous. Inappropriate

---

Case history: sense of belonging

Five medical students arrive at a distant hospital for a four week attachment. They are met by a staff member, shown around the unit, canteen, library, and accommodation. They are given name badges in the style of the existing staff, and after a couple of days are given specific roles on the unit. These roles develop over the weeks. There is little set teaching time, but the students feel free to ask any staff member for more details at quieter times.

After the attachment, they meet up with friends who were placed elsewhere. Their experience was different. No one was expecting them when they arrived, and ward and clinic staff were unhelpful. There was a set teaching programme and an enthusiastic teacher, but the students were relieved that the hospital was near a town centre with good shops and nightlife.

Case history: self esteem

A senior house officer (SHO) is making slow but steady progress. His confidence is growing and the level of supervision he requires is lessening. On one occasion, however, his case management is less than ideal, although the patient is not harmed or inconvenienced. The consultant feels exasperated and tells the SHO that everyone is carrying him and it still isn't working. The SHO subsequently reverts to seeking advice and permission for all decision making.

Students' perception of the relevance of what they are being taught is a vital motivator for learning

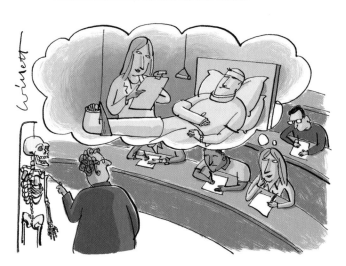

If a teacher is asked to do a one-off session with learners they don't know, he or she should prepare—both before and at the start of the session—by determining what the learners know, want to know, and expect to learn. This involves and shows respect for the learners and encourages them to invest in the session

---

Case history: role models

Dr Jones is a well known "character" in the hospital. Medical students sitting in his clinic hear him talk disparagingly about nurses, patients, and the new fangled political correctness about getting informed consent that wastes doctors' time. Most students are appalled; but a few find him engaging—they view him as a "real" doctor, unlike the ethics or communication skills lecturers.

behaviour or expression by a staff member will be noticed; at worst the learners will want to emulate that behaviour, at best they will have been given tacit permission to do so.

Maximising educational environment

Classroom, tutorials, seminars, lectures

Room temperature, comfort of seating, background noise, and visual distractions are all factors of the environment that can affect concentration and motivation. Some are within the teacher's control, others not.

Respect for the learners and their needs, praise, encouragement of participation can all lead to a positive learning experience. Lack of threat to personal integrity and self esteem is essential, although challenges can be rewarding and enjoyable.

Small group teaching facilitates individual feedback, but the seating arrangement used will have an important effect on student participation. If, for example, students sit in traditional classroom rows, those on the edges will feel excluded. A circular format encourages interaction. It allows the teacher to sit alongside a talkative person, thus keeping them out of eye contact and reducing their input. A quiet student can be placed opposite to encourage participation through non-verbal means. Students can also work in unfacilitated groups on a topic, enabling them to work in teams and share the learning tasks.

Clinical settings

In real life settings, the dual role of teacher and clinician can be complicated. The students will be closely observing the clinician, picking up hidden messages about clinical practice. They need to feel that there is no danger that they will unnecessarily distress or harm patients or their families. They also need to feel safe from humiliation. Making them feel welcomed and of value when they arrive at a new placement or post will aid their learning throughout.

Course and curriculum design

The designers of short and long courses should consider the relevance of the learning environment to the potential learners. Student representation on curriculum committees is one means of ensuring a more student centred course.

The aims, objectives, and assessments should be signposted well in advance of a course and should be demonstrably fair. The teaching methods should build on learners' experience, creating a collaborative environment. Disseminating the findings of course evaluations, followed by staff training, helps to identify and correct undesirable behaviour among faculty members. Evaluations should also include a means for reviewing the course's aims and objectives with the students.

In longer courses, student support systems and informal activities that build collective identity must be considered. Students who are having difficulties need to be identified early and given additional support.

> It is easy to "learn" attitudes—including poor attitudes. Attitudes are learnt through observation of those in relative power or seniority. Teachers must therefore be aware of providing good role modelling in the presence of students

---

Checklist to ensure good physical environment

- Is the room the right size?
- Is the temperature comfortable?
- Are there distractions (noise, visual distractions inside or outside)?
- Is the seating adequate, and how should it be arranged?
- Does the audiovisual equipment work?

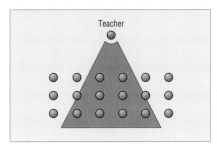

Traditional teaching can leave some students excluded (that is, outside the "triangle of influence")

Checklist for teaching in clinical settings

- Have patients and families given consent for students to be present?
- Do the staff know that teaching is planned and understand what their roles will be?
- Is there adequate space for all participants?
- How much time is available for teaching?
- How may the students be made to feel useful (for example, "pre-clerking" and presenting)?

Further reading

- Newble D, Cannon R. *A handbook for medical teachers.* 3rd ed. London: Kluwer Academic, 1994.
- Eraut M. *Developing professional knowledge and competence.* London: Falmer, 1994.
- Welsh I, Swann C. *Partners in learning: a guide to support and assessment in nurse education.* Abingdon: Radcliffe, 2002.
- Norman GR, Schmidt HG. The psychological basis of problem-based learning: a review of the evidence. *Acad Med* 1992;67:557-65.
- Dent JA, Harden RM. *A practical guide for medical teachers.* London: Churchill Livingstone, 2001.

13 Web based learning

Judy McKimm, Carol Jollie, Peter Cantillon

Many of us use the internet or the "web" (world wide web) as a source of information. In medical education, the web is increasingly used both as a learning tool to support formal programmes and as a means of delivering online learning programmes. What can educators do to ensure that the potential of the web is used effectively to support both their own learning and that of their students?

The technology

Much of the literature on web based learning shows that one of the main barriers to the effective use of teaching materials is the technology (for example, poor access, slow downloading) rather than the design of the learning materials themselves. Some of these issues are discussed later in the article, but it is vital that teachers take on expert help with technical issues in the planning, design, and delivery of web based learning programmes. Through programming and the use of "plug-ins" (programs that can be downloaded from the internet), designers can produce interactive course materials containing online activities (such as self assessments), animations, and simulations. These can improve learning and are often more enjoyable and meaningful for learners.

Distance learning

Two of the main developments in web based learning have been the adaptation of communication technology to support learning and the changes in distance learning strategies necessary for delivering online courses. Both aspects should be considered when designing or delivering web based learning programmes. Lessons can be learned by considering how distance education evolved.

Distance and open learning began with correspondence courses. The Open University in Britain is one of the best known examples of how university level education became accessible, through effective distance learning, to people who had neither the traditional qualifications nor the time to enter full time higher education.

The secret of the Open University's success lies in clearly identifying students' needs; providing effective, local support; and combining conventionally taught components with the use of up to date multimedia resources, including books, course guides, videotapes, audiotapes, television, e-conferencing, and discussion groups.

What is web based learning?

Web based learning is often called online learning or e-learning because it includes online course content. Discussion forums via email, videoconferencing, and live lectures (videostreaming) are all possible through the web. Web based courses may also provide static pages such as printed course materials.

One of the values of using the web to access course materials is that web pages may contain hyperlinks to other parts of the web, thus enabling access to a vast amount of web based information.

A "virtual" learning environment (VLE) or managed learning environment (MLE) is an all in one teaching and learning software package. A VLE typically combines functions such as

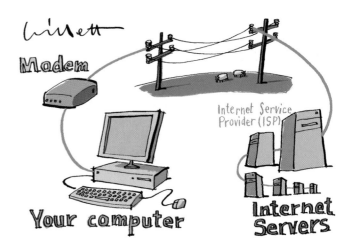

Glossary

E-conferencing—Use of online presentations and discussion forums (in real time or stored as downloadable files on a website) to avoid the need for participants to travel

E-learning—Learning through electronic means, such as via the web (see world wide web), an intranet, or other multimedia materials

HTML (hypertext markup language)—The language used to create web pages. HTML files can also contain links to other types of files including wordprocessed files, spreadsheets, presentation slides, and other web pages

Hyperlinks—Links in web pages that enable the user to access another web page (either on the same or a different site) with just one mouse click

Internet—A global network of computers divided into subsets (for example, the web or email systems). Computers are linked to the internet via host computers, which link to other computers via dial up (for example, via a modem) and network connections

Internet service provider (ISP)—Home users usually access the internet through an internet service provider (such as AOL), which maintains a network of PCs permanently connected to the internet

Intranet—A network of computers that share information, usually within an organisation. Access normally requires a password and is limited to a defined range of users

Managed learning environment (MLE)—Usually has an integrated function, providing administrative tools, such as student records, and linking with other management information systems (MLS)

Search engines (such as Lycos, Google)—Can be used to help to find information

Videostreaming—The process by which video images are able to be stored and downloaded on the web. These might be in real time (such as a conference) or used asynchronously

Virtual learning environment (VLE)—A set of electronic teaching and learning tools. Principal components include systems that can map a curriculum, track student activity, and provide online student support and electronic communication

World wide web (web)—Use of the internet to present various types of information. Websites or home pages may be accessed with the aid of a browser program (such as Netscape Communicator or Microsoft Explorer). All such programmes use HTML

For additional information see www.learnthenet.com/english/section/intbas.html

discussion boards, chat rooms, online assessment, tracking of students' use of the web, and course administration. VLEs act as any other learning environment in that they distribute information to learners. VLEs can, for example, enable learners to collaborate on projects and share information. However, the focus of web based courses must always be on the learner—technology is not the issue, nor necessarily the answer.

Models of web based learning

Several approaches can be used to develop and deliver web based learning. These can be viewed as a continuum. At one end is "pure" distance learning (in which course material, assessment, and support is all delivered online, with no face to face contact between students and teachers). At the other end is an organisational intranet, which replicates printed course materials online to support what is essentially a traditional face to face course. However, websites that are just repositories of knowledge, without links to learning, communication, and assessment activities, are not learner centred and cannot be considered true web based learning courses.

In reality, most web based learning courses are a mixture of static and interactive materials, and most ensure that some individual face to face teaching for students is a key feature of the programme.

The individual learner

The first step in designing a web based course is to identify the learners' needs and whether the learners are to be considered as part of a group or as individual learners. The web can be a useful tool for bringing isolated learners together in "virtual" groups—for example, through a discussion forum. There are several online resources on how to design web based learning programmes (for example, at www.ltsn.ac.uk).

Questions to ask before starting a web based learning project

- What is the educational purpose of the web based learning project?
- What added value will online learning bring to the course or to the students?
- What resources and expertise on web based learning exist in the institution?
- Are colleagues and the institution aware of the planned course? (You need to avoid duplication of effort and be sure that the institution's computer system can support the course)
- Has the project taken account of existing teaching resources and ongoing maintenance costs after initial development?
- Have you allowed enough time to develop or redevelop materials?
- Have the particular design and student support requirements of web based learning courses been taken into account? If not, the e-learning starter guides on the LTSN website are a good resource (www.ltsn.ac.uk/genericcentre)

Incorporating web based learning into conventional programmes

Web based learning in an institution is often integrated with conventional, face to face teaching. This is normally done via an intranet, which is usually "password protected" and accessible only to registered users. Thus it is possible to protect the intellectual property of online material and to support confidential exchange of communication between students.

Medicine has many examples of online learning, in both the basic sciences and clinical teaching. As students are usually in large groups for basic science teaching, web based learning can

> "Newer technologies such as computers and video conferencing are not necessarily better (or worse) for teaching or learning than older technologies … they are just different … The choice of technology should be driven by the needs of the learners and the context in which we are working, not by its novelty."
>
> Bates AW. *Technology, open learning and distance education.* London: Routledge, 1995

Features of a typical web based course

- Course information, notice board, timetable
- Curriculum map
- Teaching materials such as slides, handouts, articles
- Communication via email and discussion boards
- Formative and summative assessments
- Student management tools (records, statistics, student tracking)
- Links to useful internal and external websites—for example, library, online databases, and journals

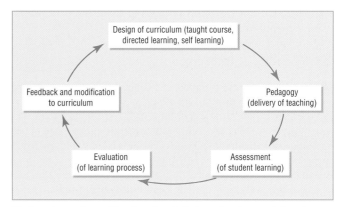

The learning cycle: useful to bear in mind when planning a web based course

Learning and teaching support network (www.ltsn.ac.uk)

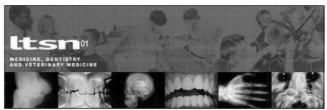

- The learning and teaching support network (consisting of 24 subject centres) was set up to help staff in higher education to deliver programmes in their own subjects more effectively and to improve communication between teachers in different organisations and government agencies
- One subject centre covers medicine, dentistry, and veterinary science (LTSN 01)
- Although not strictly web based learning, LTSN 01 uses a combination of activities delivered via the web (such as an email discussion forum, copies of useful articles, research and funding programmes, and job vacancies) to support staff working in medical, dental, and veterinary education

be used to provide learning materials to complement conventional programmes and to enable self assessment—for example, access to anatomical sites and image banks for the teaching of pathology courses. Web based learning can be useful to support clinical teaching when learners are geographically dispersed—for example, to learn clinical skills through video demonstrations.

> With web based learning, the material can be linked to libraries (for example, for ordering books or journals), online databases, and electronic journals. These functions are particularly useful for research and clinical activities

Assessment

With all types of learning, including web based learning, it is useful for students to receive constructive, timely, and relevant feedback on their progress. Online assessment is sometimes constrained by the medium in which it is operating. Computer marked assessments alone are not appropriate for marking or giving feedback on assignments such as essays or projects that require more than the mere reproduction of knowledge.

When planning online assessment it is important to determine what is to be assessed. If knowledge reproduction is being tested, objective questions (such as multiple choice or "true or false" questions) with instant or model answers can provide excellent feedback. Assessment of higher cognitive functions, such as analysis and synthesis, will require more complex tests. Automated marking may be difficult for such assessments, and the teacher is likely to have to do a substantial amount of work before he can add his or her comments to the student's record. Further guidance on how to design web based assessments for online courses can be found at www.ltsn.ac.uk and www.ltss.bris.ac.uk

For and against web based learning

When designing web based programmes (as with any learning programme), the learners' needs and experience must be taken into account. Appropriate technology and reasonable computer skills are needed to get the best out of web based or online learning. Programmes and web pages can be designed to accommodate different technical specifications and versions of software. It is frustrating for learners, however, if they are trying to work on the internet with slow access or cannot download images and videos they need. On the other hand, web based programmes may, for example, encourage more independent and active learning and are often an efficient means of delivering course materials.

Effective web teaching and learning

Course designers need to remember that younger students are more likely to be familiar with using the internet than older learners, who may feel less comfortable with a web based course. To get the best out of their learning experience, learners need basic computer skills, support, and guidance.

Teachers must design their courses to encourage effective web based learning rather than aimless "surfing." Programme design should therefore filter out poor information as well as signpost key information sources.

Many clinicians are beginning to use electronic patient records. This change means that doctors are becoming more adept at using computers and online resources to support their daily work and continuing professional development. Electronic media can facilitate access to evidence based

Advantages and disadvantages of online assessment

Advantages
- Students can receive quick feedback on their performance
- Useful for self assessments—for example, multiple choice questions
- A convenient way for students to submit assessment from remote sites
- Computer marking is an efficient use of staff time

Disadvantages
- Most online assessment is limited to objective questions
- Security can be an issue
- Difficult to authenticate students' work
- Computer marked assessments tend to be knowledge based and measure surface learning

Advantages and disadvantages of web based learning

Advantages
- Ability to link resources in many different formats
- Can be an efficient way of delivering course materials
- Resources can be made available from any location and at any time
- Potential for widening access—for example, to part time, mature, or work based students
- Can encourage more independent and active learning
- Can provide a useful source of supplementary materials to conventional programmes

Disadvantages
- Access to appropriate computer equipment can be a problem for students
- Learners find it frustrating if they cannot access graphics, images, and video clips because of poor equipment
- The necessary infrastructure must be available and affordable
- Information can vary in quality and accuracy, so guidance and signposting is needed
- Students can feel isolated

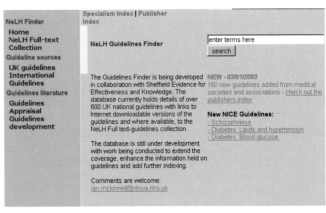

resources such as the Cochrane Library. These web based clinical support sites are excellent resources for postgraduate "on the job" learning.

Teachers should be encouraged, through training and support, to use the web and other information technologysystems in their teaching. They need examples and awareness of good practice, and standards should be set in relation to how teachers present information and manage the learning environment.

Conclusion

Web based learning offers huge opportunities for learning and access to a vast amount of knowledge and information. The role of teachers is to ensure that the learning environment provided takes account of learners' needs and ensures that they are effectively prepared and supported. Online learning has advantages, but web based learning should not always be viewed as the method of choice because barriers (such as inadequate equipment) can easily detract from student learning. The technology must therefore be applied appropriately and not used simply because it is available and new or because students and teachers have particular expectations of this means of course delivery.

Further reading

- Cook J. The role of virtual learning environments in UK medical education. *LTSN Bioscience Bulletin* 2002;5. http://bio.ltsn.ac.uk
- Forsyth I. *Teaching and learning materials and the internet.* 3rd ed. London: Kogan Page, 2001.
- Jolliffe A, Ritter J, Stevens D. *The online learning handbook: developing and using web based learning.* London: Kogan Page, 2001.
- World Federation for Medical Education. www.sund.ku.dk/WFME/ WFME%20Guidelines/guidelines99.html (paper on using information technology in education, including web based learning)

14 Creating teaching materials

Richard Farrow

The nature and qualities of the teaching materials that you use can have a substantial effect on the educational experience of your students. Teaching materials can often distract learners rather than help them to learn. Common avoidable problems include overcrowded or illegible slides, irrelevant or badly prepared handouts, and incompatible multimedia equipment. It is important therefore to know how to create effective teaching materials.

Ground rules

Five basic principles apply to preparing teaching materials, irrespective of the type of material you choose: links, intelligibility, general style, highlighting, and targeting (LIGHT). You may sometimes decide to ignore one or more of these principles, but if you do, think carefully about what you are trying to achieve.

Links
Your teaching materials should have obvious and direct links to your talk, discussion, or presentation. Handouts are the main offenders in this category, and it is not unusual for handouts to have little in common with the talk. It is quite acceptable for the teaching materials to give some additional information, but this should not be excessive.

Intelligibility
The teaching material should be easy to understand and learn from. How this is achieved will depend on the medium used and the venue of the talk or presentation. Use simple language and avoid overlong sentences or statements. Diagrams can help to clarify a complex message. If you are using slides or overhead transparencies, the size of the print needs to be large enough to be read from the back of the auditorium. The font selected should be sans serif (for example, Arial).

General style
You should aim to use a consistent style throughout your teaching materials, particularly if you are giving a series of talks. Although it is tempting to use a variety of novel styles, consistency will allow learners to concentrate on the meaning and relevance of what you are trying to communicate.

Highlighting
Highlighted information helps to emphasise important issues or pivotal points in a developing argument. Methods of highlighting include changing the colour of text or underlining words or phrases. This also applies to videotapes and audiotapes, where changing your tone of voice can be used to emphasise key points.

Targeting
It is important that both the type of educational event (for example, presentation, seminar, discussion) and the teaching materials that supplement it are targeted at what your students need to learn. Targeting therefore requires an awareness of what knowledge and skills your students already have. This can

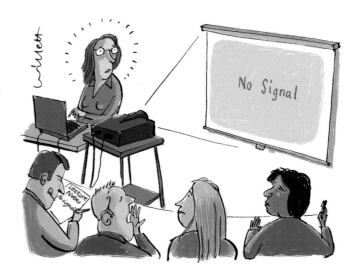

Preparing overhead transparencies

Do
- Try to use typed rather than handwritten script
- Use a type size that is big enough to be read by the whole audience—for example, at least 20 points
- Make sure that the colour of your text works—for example, dark print on a pale background
- Limit each transparency to one idea or concept

Don't
- Use small print
- Use overhead transparencies packed with tables and figures
- Use light colours

Uniformity in the teaching materials will help learners to focus on content rather than style

It is easy to **overdo** highlighting by **emphasising** virtually every point that you make. This reduces the **usefulness** of the technique and **hides** the really pivotal shifts in a *morass* of *highlighted text*.

Target your talk at learners' needs—don't just pull out the slides or overheads from a previous talk

be difficult to judge, but it is worth spending time finding out about your expected audience. It becomes easier if you are doing a series of talks with the same group as you can get feedback from the learners to help you plan more effectively.

Types of teaching materials

Black, green, or white boards
These are ideal for brainstorming sessions and small group work. If you are doing the writing, try not to talk at the same time as it is difficult for your learners to hear you if you have your back to them. Remember the LIGHT principles, and try to put concepts, not an essay, on the board. Make sure that everyone has finished copying information before you rub the board clean. Using different colours can add emphasis and highlight your important messages.

Lecture notes
Ensure that any handouts are produced to a high quality. Photocopies of handwritten notes (and frequently photocopied elderly pages) look scrappy and tend not to be valued. Give handouts to the learners at the beginning of the talk as copying down information is not a good use of their limited "face to face" time. Use headings and diagrams to make the handouts intelligible.

Overhead projector
The technical equipment for displaying overhead transparencies is widely available and reliable. It is a good backup resource, and for critical presentations it is comforting to know that, if all else fails, you have transparencies in your bag. Presentations using an overhead projector have the advantage that they allow you to face your audience while pointing out features on the transparency.

Correct preparation following the LIGHT principles is vital. Ensure that the transparencies will fit the projector—most will display A4 size, but some are smaller, so check in advance. The absolute minimum height for text on transparencies is 5 mm, although using larger text and fewer words usually produces a more effective educational tool. A good rule of thumb is to use a type size of at least 20 points. Several simple transparencies are usually better than one complicated one.

It is fairly straightforward to design your transparency on a computer then print it using a colour printer. Avoid using yellow, orange, and red, as these colours are difficult to see. Insead, use dark text on a light background. You can write and draw directly on to the transparencies with felt tipped pens. Use permanent markers to avoid smudging, and place a sheet of ruled paper underneath so that the writing is evenly spaced. You can also use a photocopier to copy print on to a transparency, but remember that you may need to enlarge it to make the text readable.

If you are likely to use a transparency again it is worth storing it carefully in dust free covers. One commonly used method is to store transparencies in clear plastic sleeves that can be filed in a ring binder. When showing transparencies, do not overuse the technique of covering the transparency and revealing a little at a time—many learners find this irritating.

35 mm slides
The need for 35 mm slides has decreased substantially with the advent of computer programs such as Microsoft's PowerPoint. However, multimedia projectors and computers are expensive and not available in all locations, whereas most educational institutions have a slide projector. Making your own slides can be difficult, so get help from the local illustration department or

Types and uses of teaching materials

Boards, flip charts—Small groups, problem based learning tutorials, workshops
Lecture notes—Small and large groups; help to improve interactivity
Overhead projector—Small and large groups, workshops, and interactive sessions
35 mm slides and PowerPoint—Generally large groups and lecture formats
Videos—Good for clinical teaching in larger groups (use film of patients); also for teaching communication skills and practical skills (students can keep films for self appraisal)
Life and plastic models—Anatomy teaching in small groups or for self directed learning
Computer assisted learning packages—Small groups with a tutor; large groups in computer laboratories; self directed learning
Skills centres and simulators—Small groups learning clinical skills

Leave spaces in the handout for your learners to record the results of interactive parts of your talk—this ensures that the handout the learners take away has more value than the one they were given. Also, leave spaces for exercises to be completed later, thus linking self directed learning with face to face learning

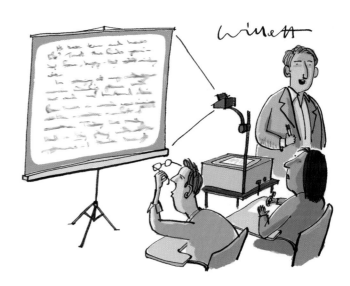

Paper copies of transparencies and slides can make useful handouts—your learners can then add clarifying statements or diagrams to their own copy of the presentation

Number your slides so that if a projectionist is loading them or the carousel is dropped they can be quickly reordered

a commercial company. Ensure that the text is large enough to see when projected and that the slides are marked so that they are loaded in the projector correctly. Dual projection is rarely done well and rarely necessary unless you are using visual images (for example, *x* ray films, clinical photographs) with accompanying text. If you use dual projection make sure that each of the slides is labelled for the correct projector.

Computer generated slides

The ability to make computer generated slides (for example, PowerPoint) has transformed the way that many people create teaching materials and has greatly reduced the use of 35 mm slides. Try not to get seduced by the technology, however, and remember that it is just another educational tool. Having tried all of the colours and slide layouts available, many experienced lecturers now prefer simple formats that are easy to read and in which the medium does not get in the way of the message.

However, the computer package has many useful tools—diagrams and "clip art" can help to conceptualise difficult problems. Video clips can be inserted into a presentation, but be certain that they are there to illustrate a point and not simply to show off your own technological skills. Use advanced formats for PowerPoint presentations only if you are well practised and comfortable with the medium.

Ensure that the computer you are planning to use is compatible with the multimedia projector. Similarly, if you have stored your presentation on a CD or floppy disk (or any one of the other portable storage formats), make sure that this is supported at the venue. The latest version of the presentation software can give you access to many features that may not work on the computer provided at the teaching venue, so a wise precaution is to save your presentation as an older version of the software.

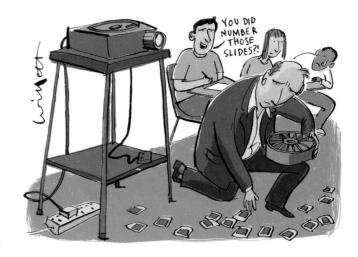

Ground rules for slide preparation (35 mm or PowerPoint)
- Use a clear font that is easily readable
- Use a type size of 20 points or greater
- Use a light text on a dark background for slides (in contrast with OHP transparencies)
- Use short sentences and small tables
- Restrict the overall number of words on each slide to about 40 or fewer
- Avoid patterned backgrounds—they are extremely distracting
- Limit the number of colours on your slides to a maximum of three
- Use highlighting to emphasise items in lists
- Use animation and sound effects sparingly

Further reading

- Cannon R, Newble D. *A handbook for teachers in universities and colleges.* 4th ed. London: Kogan Page, 1999.
- Newble DI, Cannon R. *A handbook for medical teachers.* 4th ed. Dordrecht, Netherlands: Kluwer Academic, 2001.
- Kemp JE, Dayton DK. *Planning and producing instructional media.* 5th ed. New York: Harper and Row, 1985.
- Hartley J. *Designing instructional text.* 3rd ed. London: Kogan Page, 1994.

Index

Index

The complete ABC series

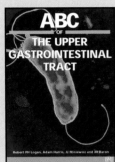

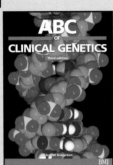

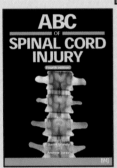

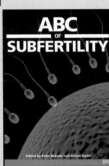

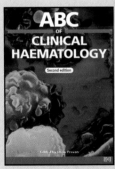